D0745756

Social inequalities in health
New evidence and policy implications

Social inequalities in health
New evidence and policy implications

Edited by

Johannes Siegrist and
Michael Marmot

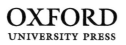

OXFORD
UNIVERSITY PRESS

OXFORD
UNIVERSITY PRESS

Great Clarendon Street, Oxford OX2 6DP

Oxford University Press is a department of the University of Oxford.
It furthers the University's objective of excellence in research, scholarship,
and education by publishing worldwide in

Oxford New York

Auckland Cape Town Dar es Salaam Hong Kong Karachi
Kuala Lumpur Madrid Melbourne Mexico City Nairobi
New Delhi Shanghai Taipei Toronto

With offices in

Argentina Austria Brazil Chile Czech Republic France Greece
Guatemala Hungary Italy Japan Poland Portugal Singapore
South Korea Switzerland Thailand Turkey Ukraine Vietnam

Oxford is a registered trade mark of Oxford University Press
in the UK and in certain other countries

Published in the United States
by Oxford University Press Inc., New York

British Library Cataloguing in Publication Data

Data available

Library of Congress Cataloging in Publication Data

Data available

Typeset by Newgen Imaging Systems (P) Ltd., Chennai, India
Printed in Great Britain
on acid-free paper by
Biddles Ltd., King's Lynn, Norfolk

ISBN 978-0-19-856816-2

Preface

The contributions of this book result from a scientific programme, Social Variations in Health Expectancy in Europe, which was funded by the European Science Foundation (ESF) from 1999 to 2003. This initiative aimed at advancing the most recent promising research developments in this field by strengthening scientific collaboration throughout Europe. Impressive achievements were obtained as a result of a series of scientific meetings, conferences, training courses and exchange of scientists between research centres (see Chapter 1). The selection of the following chapters, while not representing all major results, highlights the topical importance of main work areas in this programme, and it illustrates particularly promising scientific advances.

We are grateful to all participants of the ESF Programme, and especially to the authors of the chapters of this book, for their seminal contributions. Our special thanks are due to the Standing Committee for the Social Sciences and the European Medical Research Council, two ESF research councils which, for the first time, coordinated their efforts to initiate and realize this programme. We acknowledge the excellent support provided by Simone Weyers, M.A., University of Duesseldorf whose efforts were essential in preparing this book. We also thank Ruth Bell, Ph.D., University College London for her editorial assistance and Oxford University Press for a very productive cooperation.

The Editors

Contents

Contributors

Lisa F. Berkman
Department of Society,
Human Development and Health,
Harvard School of Public Health,
Boston, MA USA.

Hans Bosma
Department of Medical Sociology,
Maastricht University,
Maastricht,
The Netherlands.

Espen Dahl
Oslo University College,
Norway.

Johan Fritzell
Centre for Health Equity Studies,
Stockholm University/Karolinska
Institutet,
Sweden.

Margareta Kristenson
Department of Health and Society,
Linköping University,
Sweden.

Diana Kuh
Medical Research Council National
Survey of Health and Development,
Department of Epidemiology and
Public Health, Royal Free and
University College London
Medical School,
London, UK.

Anton Kunst
Department of Public Health,
Erasmus MC,

University Medical Center
Rotterdam,
The Netherlands.

Eero Lahelma
Department of Public Health,
University of Helsinki,
Finland.

Frank J. van Lenthe
Department of Public Health,
Erasmus MC,
University Medical Center
Rotterdam,
The Netherlands.

Johan P. Mackenbach
Department of Public Health,
Erasmus MC,
University Medical Center
Rotterdam,
The Netherlands.

Michael Marmot
International Centre for
Health and Society,
University College London,
London, UK.

Pekka Martikainen
Department of Sociology,
University of Helsinki,
Finland.

Maria Melchior
Institut National
de la Santé de la Recherche Médicale,
Saint-Maurice Cedex,
France.

Chris Power
Centre for Paediatric
Epidemiology and Biostatistics,
Institute of Child Health,
University College London,
London, UK.

Johannes Siegrist
Department of Medical
Sociology,
Medical Faculty,
University of Duesseldorf,
Germany.

Andrew Steptoe
Department of Epidemiology
and Public Health,
University College London,
London, UK.

Töres Theorell
National Institute for
Psychosocial Factors
and Health,
Stockholm,
Sweden.

Chapter 1

Introduction

Johannes Siegrist and Michael Marmot

Social inequalities in health: basic facts

> Lower socio-economic status is probably the most
> powerful single contributor to premature morbidity
> and mortality, not only in the United States, but
> worldwide.
> (*Williams* 1998)

While socially determined health inequalities have been reported since the early
stages of industrialization of western societies, and particularly by pioneers such
as Chadwick, Villermé and Virchow, a widespread belief assumed that health
inequalities would be disappearing in contemporary modern societies. For
instance, in the 1960s, an American scholar concluded that 'in modern western
countries the relationship between social class and the prevalence of illness is
certainly decreasing and most probably no longer exists' (Kadushin 1964). Yet,
as mentioned, at the turn of the twenty-first century, social inequalities in health
continue to be a key public health problem in advanced societies, including
European countries.

With the development of social epidemiology and medical sociology,
evidence of strong variations in life expectancy between and within countries
has accumulated over the past three or four decades (Townsend and Davidson
1982, Elstad 2000, Fox 1989, Kunst 1997, Mackenbach and Bakker 2002,
Marmot and Wilkinson 2006). With regard to mortality, mean difference in
life expectancy between those at the top and at the bottom of a society's social
structure (as defined by education, income, employment status) are anywhere
from four to ten years. For instance, in Finland, life expectancy at age 35 for
men employed in white-collar jobs was 6.9 years higher than that of manual
workers in 1995 (Lahelma 2001). Marked socio-economic differences are
reported in the United Kingdom (Drever and Whitehead 1997), the United States
(Pappas *et al.* 1993), Sweden, France, the Netherlands, Norway, Denmark,
Czech Republic and Hungary (Kunst 1997, Mackenbach *et al.* 1997, Valkonen
et al. 1997). In Switzerland, a recent study documented a mean difference in
life expectancy at birth of 4.4 years between men in the highest and in the

lowest social stratum (Gubéran and Usel 2000). Several epidemiological investigations observed a widening of social inequalities in health during the final quarter of the last century (Fox 1989, Marmot and McDowall 1986, Drever and Whitehead 1997). In view of considerable progress in medical science, constant increase in health care spending and extension of health care facilities, this observation is particularly challenging.

There has, rightly, been much concern with the effects of material deprivation accounting for the worse health of the poor compared to that of those not in poverty. This is a partial picture. The problem of inequality in health is not confined to the poorest members of society, but there is a social gradient of mortality and morbidity across the whole of a society. With each step one moves up on the social ladder, the better one's health. The explanations for this social gradient in health have been the focus of the Whitehall studies (Marmot *et al.* 1978, Marmot 2004), although the observation had been there in the literature before Whitehall defined it as a major object of study (Antonovsky 1967, Kitagawa and Hauser 1973). For instance, findings from the first Whitehall study of British Civil Servants show that, at younger ages, men in the lowest (office support) employment grades have a four times higher mortality rate than men in the highest administrative grade. As striking as the difference between the top and bottom is the gradient. Position in the hierarchy shows a strong correlation with mortality risk. Men second from the top have higher mortality than top-grade civil servants; clerical officers have higher mortality rates than the men above them in hierarchy. A social gradient was seen not only for total mortality, but for all the major causes of death, including coronary heart disease and stroke (Marmot *et al.* 1984, van Rossum *et al.* 2000). Moreover, as documented in the Whitehall II study, several important risk factors of chronic degenerative diseases follow this social gradient (Marmot *et al.* 1991).

The social gradient of health confronts current research with several challenges. First, the gradient varies across the life course where it is steepest at two stages, early childhood and midlife. Less inequality is observed in adolescence and in older age (Kuh and Ben Shlomo 2004). Second, there are important gender differences. Among men, the gradient is steeper than among women (Arber and Thomas 2001). Third, important variations in size of inequality have been documented across countries, even within relatively homogenous economic regions, such as western European countries (Kunst 1997, Mackenbach *et al.* 1997). A fourth variation concerns the health measure under study. A striking feature of the social gradient in health has been that it cuts across specific medical conditions; there are, however, exceptions. In general, morbidity and mortality differences are pronounced in highly prevalent chronic diseases and disorders, such as cardiovascular diseases, depression, suicide and other violent deaths, type 2 diabetes and other obesity related disorders, lung cancer, respiratory disorders, liver cirrhosis, and sexually transmitted diseases (van Rossum *et al.* 2000). Less pronounced differences are observed in other types of cancer, gastrointestinal diseases, and neurological disorders, among others, whereas a small number of diseases follow the opposite social gradient: the higher the social status, the higher the prevalence (e.g. breast cancer, asthma).

Finally, health inequalities vary according to the measure of social status under study. This represents an opportunity rather than a problem. Most frequently used measures of social status are employment or occupational class, education, and income. Although interrelated, these measures of social inequality point to different phenomena. By taking a theoretically grounded approach to measurement of social position potential light can be shed on causal mechanisms. As social position might represent differences in level of deprivation, in social standing, and in power, different indicators are needed to measure these aspects. This argument is of special relevance when social inequalities according to gender are studied. For instance, Sacker and collegues (2000) have shown similar inequalities in health for men and women, but interesting differences in the way these are best demonstrated. A socio-economic measure that reflects the nature of the job best predicts the social gradient in mortality in men, whereas a measure that reflects general social standing best predicts the social gradient in women.

Rather than simply compare the predictive power of different measures, the researcher can now ask how well these measures represent different features of socio-economic position. In addition to theory there are practical considerations. Education as a measure has the advantage that it avoids the problem of health-related social mobility later in life, i.e., although ill-health developing, say, in middle age could lead to drop in income and affect employment prospects – and thereby lead to a relation between ill-health and low social position – this does not apply to education which is completed before ill-health in midlife starts. A second practical consideration is that although occupational characteristics cover most relevant aspects of socio-economic inequalities, their application is limited to employed populations (Krieger *et al.* 1997, Lahelma 2001). In addition to using these measures of social status separately, summary indices combining the three variables are sometimes applied. This area of measurement is further complicated by the fact that social structures change over time, that the significance of these indicators may change (e.g. between 'materialist' and 'postmaterialist' societies), and that new types of social differentiation within populations may emerge.

In summary, there are solid facts demonstrating a social gradient of morbidity and mortality in modern societies with those at the bottom of the ladder having poorer health than those in the middle and those at the top. However, variations of this gradient are observed according to stage of the life course, gender, type of country, indicator of health and indicator of social inequality under study. In view of these challenges the search for explanations of the social gradient and its variations is a most important task. This book reports on significant progress in solving this task. It discusses new explanations and explores their implications for policy measures that aim at reducing health disparities. These explanations differ from the answers that were traditionally given to this question. Therefore, let us first consider briefly these traditional answers before outlining the aims and contents of this book.

Traditional explanations of the social gradient

A major effort towards explaining social inequalities in health was provided by the Black Report in the United Kingdom (Townsend and Davidson 1982) and the debates following the publication of this report (Davey Smith *et al.* 1990, MacIntyre 1997). The importance of the Black Report was in highlighting inequalities in health as a scientific and policy issue, in giving focus to the problem, and in providing a framework for discussion on causes of inequalities. It had a huge effect on the field of research and led directly to a second UK scientific and policy review, the Acheson Report (Acheson 1998). The explanatory framework provided by Black shaped the discussion for two decades. As we shall show, the discussion and research questions have now moved to a new level. Distinctions that Black made, for example, between material and cultural explanations are now shown by later research not to be clear cut. Material conditions can have important influences on culture and behaviour.

Underlying these efforts was a discussion about terminology and policy implications. Basically, four different terms are used in this context: 'social variations in health', 'social disparities in health', 'social inequalities in health', and 'social inequities in health'. In the first two cases, health differences between population groups are described without referring to a principle of vertical social stratification, i.e. core scarce resources that are unequally distributed across the hierarchy of social status positions available within a society. This latter is the case with the term 'social inequalities' which addresses the differences in power and resources that are related to socio-economic status. Yet all three terms lack an explicit reference to the normative principle of social justice. The use of these former terms is preferred in official reports and policy documents that tend to avoid implications involving injustice (e.g. Agency for Healthcare Research and Quality 2003).

In contrast, 'inequities in health' are considered unfair and unjust to the extent that they are avoidable. Equity in health means that everyone has fair opportunity to attain their full health potential. As such, equity is fundamental to the mission of improving population health (Krieger 2005). Social gradients of health contradict the basic principle of 'fair equality of opportunity' of fundamental human life chances (Daniels 1996, Rawls 2001). Thus, knowledge about their causes calls for policies to reduce them. In this perspective, research on social inequities in health is a prerequisite for, and an important part of, health policy action at different levels of impact (regional, national, international).

Although we subscribe to this view we nevertheless prefer to use the term 'social inequalities' instead of 'social inequities'. The main reason is that our current state of knowledge does not allow us to make definite judgments about 'avoidable' and 'unavoidable' disease conditions as we certainly need to extend our knowledge on the web of causation of major chronic diseases and the extent to which they are socially determined.

The Black Report proposed four types of explanation that are only partly exclusive: (1) artefact, (2) natural or social selection, (3) materialist or structuralist, and (4) cultural or behavioural explanations. The artefact explanation claims that the observed association between social status and health is spurious, largely due to measurement error of the variables under study. The plausibility of this explanation may be restricted to official administrative data with recognized problems of numerator/denominator according to census data and death certificates. The argument is not applicable to longitudinal observational studies with individual data (from which substantial evidence is derived).

The natural or social selection explanation posits that health determines social position, i.e. that health 'selects' people into different social strata. As poor health leads to lower position in the social hierarchy, the direction of causation is completely reversed. Again, longitudinal investigations, preferably birth cohort studies, allow a test of the direction of causality. Available evidence suggests that the contribution of poor health during childhood on social mobility later in life is real, but small, and that the causal direction is likely to be from social environment to illness, not the other way. However, as will be demonstrated in Chapter 2, a dynamic conceptualization of the interaction between 'nature' and 'nurture' provides new insights into the interdependence of biological (largely genetic) with social influences on health. It is of interest to consider 'indirect' genetic selection as a potentially relevant determinant of the social gradient of health, as recently suggested by Mackenbach (2005). For instance, given a strong genetic impact on intelligence, one could argue that intelligence is a driving force of socially upward mobility which, therefore, to some extent results from indirect genetic selection (Nettle 2003). It is, of course, important to make the distinction between the explanations for why an individual reaches a certain socio-economic position, and why occupation of that position leads to a given risk of illness (Marmot 2004). For example, intelligence, in part determined by genetic endowment, may influence attained social position in adult life. It may not, however, be the level of intelligence that is related to risk of illness, but the circumstances attached to attained social position.

The materialist or structuralist explanation claims that material resources related to income and occupational position (which are both largely influenced by education) have a direct impact on health. As income determines a wide range of life circumstances one can assume that conditions such as poor housing, cheap and unhealthy food, lack of safety measures, or exposure to occupational hazards all contribute to poor health. These effects are not confined to exposed people, but are transmitted to offspring through transgenerational chains of deprivation. MacIntyre (1997) has pointed out that this is a narrow interpretation of 'materialist'. A softer version would include psychosocial factors. Although some suppose that materialist approaches exclude psychosocial factors (Lynch *et al.* 2000), there is no reason why this should be so (Marmot and Wilkinson 2001). An exclusive emphasis on the physical life circumstances associated with low income fails to recognize the importance of a broad spectrum of psychosocial influences on health that interact with material conditions and that may be decisive in explaining the social gradient among populations with standards of living above a certain threshold of poverty and deprivation. In fact, large parts of this book illustrate and support this argument.

According to the fourth explanation health-related lifestyles account for social inequalities in morbidity and mortality. To a large extent, cultural influences shape health-damaging and health-promoting behaviour through processes of socialization that are socially graded. Poor diet, smoking, alcohol consumption, lack of physical exercise and overweight are more prevalent in lower socio-economic status groups. At the same time, these behaviours act as powerful determinants of major chronic diseases, and this fact explains much of their socially graded distribution across society. There is no doubt about the significance of this well-established argument, yet it does not help in explaining why people in less advantaged life circumstances display these behaviours more often than people who are better off.

More recently, it was suggested to integrate this fourth explanation offered by the Black Report into a broader perspective of sociocultural shaping of individual behaviour by referring to Bourdieu's concept of 'habitus' (Singh-Manoux and Marmot 2005). According to Bourdieu (1993), the term 'habitus' points to the correspondence between sociostructural opportunities or constraints and practices of everyday life in different domains. Through the processes of socialization, these practices come to be embodied as schemes of perceiving, feeling and acting, thus giving rise to characteristic dispositions of behaviour that are transmitted from one generation to the next. 'Habitus' or the structure–disposition–practice scheme is not restricted to health behaviours, but extends to the acquisition of cognitive, motivational and interpersonal skills that are crucial for personal development and for coping with adversities in life. Thus, social positions create socialized dispositions among individuals who grow up in respective sociocultural environments and who acquire these dispositions through processes of observation, imitation and internalization.

We can derive three conclusions from this short discussion of traditional explanations of the social gradient of health, as suggested by the Black Report. First, as mentioned, these explanations are not mutually exclusive. Rather they underline the complexities of causation when dealing with social determinants of health. An exclusive emphasis on one particular type of explanation runs the risk of bypassing essential interactions of social structure with individual behaviour. Second, although labelled 'traditional' some of these explanations are open to promising extensions and new interpretations. For instance, we mentioned the role of genetic susceptibility as a means of producing indirect social selection. With the advent of a series of new research findings on 'gene $\times$ environment' interactions, this approach will merit careful attention in future research. Another example of extension concerns research on health-related lifestyles, in particular its link with a sociological perspective of socialized dispositions that are analysed as class-specific habitus. Third, it became obvious that a broad range of psychosocial phenomena with relevance to the social gradient of health are neglected in this typology of explanations, at the expense of an overly favoured material explanation.

This latter conclusion has been an essential motivation to produce this book. Obviously, the editors' motivation was shared by a larger network of scientists engaged in research on social inequalities in health. Hence, the activities of this network and the production of the following chapters emanating from it need to be described.

New evidence: a scientific programme of the European Science Foundation

The aims and structure of the Programme

The past 25 years of social epidemiological research on health inequalities have provided basic tools, standardized methods and rich empirical evidence. As was mentioned, comparative analyses on socio-economic differences in mortality and morbidity in Europe revealed a consistent pattern of a stepwise increased risk according to lower educational and occupational standing. Building on the achievements of this seminal research, it was increasingly felt by researchers that the next major task of science consists in moving from description to explanation and, by doing so, to extend the types of previously proposed explanations. Substantial recent progress along three separate lines of research has reinforced this perspective:

1 The availability of data from longitudinal (and, in particular, birth cohort) studies, that demonstrate the dynamic interaction of biologic with socio-economic and psychosocial factors in a life course perspective;

2 The design and successful testing of theoretical models that seek to explain social variations in exposure to stressful living and working environments and their adverse effects on health;

3 Progress in multi-level analysis of large data sets which link information on the macro-social environment (e.g. income inequality, labour market dynamics, participation in social capital) with variations in morbidity and mortality.

Each year, the European Science Foundation (ESF), an organization of national research councils of European countries, calls for applications of a limited number of scientific programmes to be funded by its members. Scientific programmes are intended to advance the state of research in areas considered to be of outstanding relevance to Europe. Rather than supporting original research of scientists within or between single countries, this programme is intended to strengthen research collaboration throughout Europe by funding a series of structured scientific meetings and conferences, by enabling exchange of investigators between the research centres, by organizing training courses and summer schools, and by promoting joint scientific publications. In 1999, a joint application of a scientific programme on Social Variations in Health Expectancy in Europe was successful and was sponsored for a five year period (Siegrist and Weyers 2004).

For the first time, two ESF research councils, the Standing Committee for the Social Sciences and the European Medical Research Council, coordinated their efforts to support a scientific programme that aims at advancing explanations of one of the most urgent and well-documented modern public health problems, the widening of social inequalities in morbidity and mortality between and within countries. This programme has been supported by 22 ESF Member Organizations of 13 European countries, and it has assembled some 70 scientists from Europe including a transatlantic link with leading researchers from the United States and Canada. Collaborative work was largely organized along three topics dealt with in three respective working groups.

The focus of Work Group I was on life course approaches towards explaining social inequalities in health, with particular emphasis on early life. Life course perspectives on health and health inequalities represent a new field of research on health and health inequalities. Perspectives which recognize that individual well-being is shaped by processes operating over the course of life ('the life course') have long been central to other research fields, including psychology and sociology, but these perspectives are only beginning to assume the same centrality in social epidemiology, bringing to the discipline a greater appreciation of how people's health is influenced by biological and social factors acting over time and across generations – and how differential exposure to these factors contributes to inequalities in health (Kuh and Ben-Shlomo 2004). Both across Europe and internationally, the development of life course epidemiology is stimulating new conceptual and methodological approaches which bridge the social and biological sciences and which bring research closer to policy. Understanding the life course influences on adult health requires a focus on the different and changing environments in which children grow up and adults grow older. An eco-social perspective is thus integral to a life course perspective, with studies seeking to track risk factors operating at range of hierarchical levels – from the macro-social, through the meso-social environments of home, workplace and community, to the individual and molecular level.

The research agenda outlined for the Working Group focused on areas in which members could best make a contribution to the enhancement and scientific transfer of life course perspectives in Europe. Three areas were identified, and the objectives of the Working Group were given priority accordingly:

- to pool the skills of the group to tackle conceptual and methodological issues central to life course analyses;
- to exploit the potential of established datasets to investigate questions about life course influences on health and health inequalities;
- to take the opportunity presented by new cohort studies to establish dialogue and, if possible, cross-linkages between them.

Work Group II concentrated on social and psychological determinants of health in midlife and on psychobiological pathways linking an adverse psychosocial environment with ill health. A psychosocial environment was defined as the sociostructural range of opportunities that is available to an individual person to meet his or her needs of well-being, productivity and positive self-experience, in particular self-efficacy and self-esteem (Siegrist and Marmot 2004). These opportunities are available through the acquisition and maintenance of core social roles in adult life, such as the marital and family roles, the work role, and civic roles. Given the centrality of work and employment for well-being and health in adult life, and particularly in midlife, the research agenda developed in this Working Group put special emphasis on the contribution of innovative analyses of an adverse psychosocial work environment towards explaining health inequalities. Its main objectives were:

- to advance explanations of social inequalities in health across Europe by focusing on theoretical models that identify adverse psychosocial environments and by testing their impact on health;
- to advance the development of standardized measures of stressful psychosocial environments across Europe and to initiate comparative data analysis;
- to develop new psychobiological markers of stress and to apply them to population subgroups that are exposed to psychosocial adversity.

Two such theoretical models received special attention: the demand–control model and the effort–reward imbalance model (see below). They were both developed within the context of work–stress-related research, but have been applied to other types of adverse psychosocial environments more recently. As several epidemiological investigations in Europe collected data on these models through standardized measures, the time has come to conduct comparative data analysis within this Working Group (for a summary of results see Marmot and Siegrist 2004). Some of these epidemiological studies, notably the Whitehall II study and several Swedish studies, offered opportunities of including established and new psychobiological markers of stress in subgroups, thus creating fresh evidence on mechanisms that possibly mediate an adverse psychosocial environment with reduced health.

In Working Group III, the main interest was on studying the effects of the macro-social environment on health, and more specifically to study its contribution to the explanation of socio-economic inequalities in health. It has been increasingly recognized that a focus on more 'proximal' explanatory factors may conceal important influences from more 'distal' determinants of morbidity and mortality. Thus, macro-social contexts are to be brought back into public health research, in particular with the advent of new statistical tools of conducting multi-level analysis (Diez-Roux 1998). Two such contextual factors received special attention: income inequality and aggregate neighbourhood deprivation.

The aims of the Working Group were:

- to discuss conceptual and methodological challenges of research on income inequality and health;

- to carry out a comparative study of associations between income and health in several European countries;
- to improve the methodology of measuring aggregate neighbourhood deprivation and to carry out a comparative study on its association with mortality.

Furthermore, as social inequalities in health in western Europe seem to be as large in more 'egalitarian' countries as in the less 'egalitarian' ones, an additional aim of this Working Group consisted in studying the influence of different types of welfare regimes (e.g. 'social-democratic' versus 'liberal') on health disparities in respective countries.

In summary, the aims of this Scientific Programme were:

- advancing explanations in the three research clusters of Working Groups I, II, and III which hold special promise for scientific progress;
- strengthening transdisciplinary collaboration between biomedical and social science research teams (especially Working Groups I and II);
- developing a strong science transfer component across Europe, including the creation of scientific networks as well as recruitment and involvement of young scholars;
- contributing to health policy activities at the European and national level by informing responsible agencies and bodies about major research results and their implications, e.g. for the design and implementation of preventive measures.

The following chapters represent essential achievements obtained from the activities within the three Working Groups of this Scientific Programme. While the selection of the contributions is far from being representative of a very productive scientific output that resulted in a large number of scientific papers, as indicated in the Final Report (Siegrist and Weyers 2004), it nevertheless reflects the topical importance of the main work conducted within these networks.

In the following section, the reader is given a short summary of each chapter. The final section of this introduction discusses future challenges to this field of research and to the transfer of its findings into health policy.

Content of the book

Chris Power and Diana Kuh played a major role in guiding and developing the scientific activities of Working Group I. With their chapter Life course development of unequal health they provide a highly remarkable contribution to the current state of research on exposures during early stages of life and their influence on adult health. Starting with an identification of those factors from early and later life stages that are implicated in the development of adult disease, Power and Kuh first show to what extent these factors are socially patterned. Prominent examples of social patterning are poor growth *in utero*, postnatal weight gain, childhood height, and exposure to tobacco. Following this, selective evidence on effects of the social environment in early life on adult inequalities in risk behaviour, morbidity and mortality is presented, drawing on results from British birth cohort studies and additional sources. Results clearly indicate that those from manual origins exhibited elevated risks of morbidity and mortality during midlife, even after adjusting for the effects of adult socio-economic position. However, the strength of these effects varies according to the disease condition under study. Third, the authors discuss why it is important to consider health and functional trajectories as well as the more conventional outcomes of morbidity and mortality in life course approaches towards health inequalities. These former outcomes are better suited to capture developmental health in terms of health capital and health potential. Power and Kuh present a conceptual framework that outlines how developmental health is affected by an adverse early social environment and the 'chains of risk' it may elicit in later periods. This illuminating framework is illustrated with original findings on (1) unequal development of psychological distress and self-rated poor health, (2) contribution of childhood growth and lifetime weight gain to the unequal development of coronary heart disease, and (3) contribution of neurodevelopmental factors to adult health. Furthermore, the authors discuss socially different functional decline in midlife and its significance in predicting disability and death later on, and they show the impact of early life on functional trajectories. In summary, this chapter is both an inspiring account of conceptual approaches to life course analysis of the social gradient of disease, and a demonstration and discussion of a series of impressive recent research findings obtained from birth cohort studies.

In their chapter on social integration, family structure and population health Lisa F. Berkman and Maria Melchior demonstrate the fruitfulness of a transatlantic scientific collaboration that was in part supported by the ESF Programme. Building on her classic Alameda county study on social integration and mortality (Berkman and Syme 1979), Harvard scientist Berkman, together with French psychologist Melchior, test this association in a large longitudinal data set on male and female employees in France, the GAZEL study. Their results indicate that the risk of all-cause mortality is clearly associated with level of social integration. There is a steady gradient in risk with decreasing social connections. When exploring the specific causes of death, findings (restricted to men for reasons of statistical power) show a steep gradient for cancer mortality and a significant association with accidents or suicide. However, contrary to the findings from several US studies, cardiovascular mortality was unrelated to social integration in France. What makes this chapter unique is the authors' attempt to link these comparative epidemiological findings with structural and economic conditions that determine opportunities of social integration within respective countries, i.e. France and the United States. Differences in family and relationship-friendly policies and in immigration policies between the two countries are discussed. They indicate more family-friendly programmes as well as more intense social exchange within social networks in France although their potential health benefit cannot be assessed by available data. In their final part authors refer to the possible gain of intervention studies. While micro-social modifications of social networks have had only modest impacts on health these effects might possibly be larger if such interventions modify social policies. It goes unsaid that lower socio-economic status groups would profit most from such interventions because their opportunities of experiencing work- and family-friendly living arrangements are particularly restricted.

As mentioned above, quality of work is important for health and well-being, but it is also socially graded across employed populations. Therefore, analysing associations of work, socio-economic position and health may offer new insights into the ways in which adverse psychosocial environments 'get under the skin' to produce poor health and disease. The chapter by Johannes Siegrist and Töres Theorell sets out to explore the role of work and employment in explaining health inequalities, one of the central aims of Working Group II of the ESF Programme. Their analysis starts with the description of two prominent theoretical models of identifying an adverse psychosocial work environment, the demand–control model and the effort–reward imbalance model. Both authors made substantial contributions to the development of these concepts (Karasek and Theorell 1990, Siegrist 1996). The demand–control model posits that stressful experience at work depends on a specific job task profile characterized by high quantitative demands in combination with low control. Low control at work is defined as limited decision latitude and as lack of skill discretion. The effort–reward imbalance model is rooted in the general principle of social reciprocity in contractual exchange. It claims that high efforts spent at work that are not met by adequate rewards (money, esteem, promotion prospects, job security) elicit recurrent stressful experience. This imbalance is likely to occur in people who have no alternative choice or are in highly competitive jobs. Personal coping (overcommitment) is important as well. Results of epidemiological and naturalistic studies supporting the models are presented and discussed, including effects on health produced by macroeconomic context of work stress (globalization). A further paragraph is devoted to an elucidation of the relationship between social inequalities, quality of work in terms of the two models and health, whereas the final section discusses policy implications of current evidence in this important field of inequality research.

Based on his long-standing research on psychobiological stress mechanisms, Andrew Steptoe addresses the crucial question of how variations in socio-economic position affect the organism by means of enhanced stress responses. Following McEwen's (1998) concept of allostasis, Steptoe first discusses findings from laboratory mental stress testing that give some indication of greater stress reactivity or slower post-stress recovery among participants with low socio-economic status. The Whitehall II Study offers opportunities to compare differences in acute stress responses and post-stress recovery of cardiovascular and haemostatic measures between lower and higher status groups. More specifically, greater increase in plasma interleukin-6 and less effective post-stress recovery in cardiovascular reactivity and in plasma viscosity is found in lower grade participants. This approach is further validated in naturalistic studies of physiological activity in everyday life where multiple measures of cardiovascular activity and salivary cortisol are available. One of the interesting findings indicates higher systolic blood pressure over the working day in lower status civil servants with a high level of work-related overcommitment. This may mirror an experience of recurrent goal frustration in a job that lacks any promotion prospects. Steptoe's research must be considered a particularly promising approach towards unravelling the 'hidden injuries of social class'.

While the main focus of the former chapters is on differential exposure according to socio-economic position, the next two chapters deal with differential coping of exposed people. Margareta Kristenson starts her contribution with a distinction between coping strategies and coping abilities. The former describe ways of appraising and dealing with challenges and threats, whereas the latter refers to the expectancies and experiences of people's internal resources. More specifically, coping ability is contingent on the strength of positive outcome expectancy which in turn reinforces coping strategies. On the other hand, lack of positive outcome expectancy induces feelings of helplessness. According to Kristenson, children from a lower socio-economic background have fewer opportunities of developing positive outcome expectancies during socialization than those with a more privileged background. To some extent, these group differences in coping ability may account for differential susceptibility to socioenvironmental stressors in adult life and greater vulnerability in terms of stress-related disorders. Results from a psychobiological study provide some support of this latter hypothesis. In two groups of middle-aged men in Lithuania and Sweden, a significant association was found between socio-economic position and positive outcome expectancy. Moreover, the pattern of stress reactivity (cortisol response) to a standardized mental challenge varied according to social status and outcome expectancy: men with low status and negative outcome expectancy displayed significantly elevated baseline levels of cortisol while the responsiveness of cortisol during challenge was compromised. These findings, together with those reported by Steptoe, are of interest because they are among the first to link socio-economic status and health with psychobiological mechanisms that are implicated in the development of chronic diseases.

The concepts of coping ability and control belief overlap quite substantially, as documented in Hans Bosma's chapter on socio-economic differences in control beliefs. These latter refer to assumptions about personal influence on life circumstances. People with low socio-economic status often react with fatalism to challenges as they lack a strong belief in their mastery. Low control beliefs are transmitted through socialization and reinforced by adverse working and living conditions. They predispose low status people to elevated risks of depression and health-adverse behaviours. Moreover, stress-induced neuroendocrine and immunological pathways may be implicated (see the chapters by Steptoe and Kristenson). Bosma presents new data indicating that the contribution of control beliefs to the association of social status with another prevalent disorder, coronary heart disease, is substantial. In a follow-up study of Dutch men and women in early old age about one-third of the socio-economic differences in disease occurrence can be attributed to control beliefs. Even stronger effects are seen in another prospective study, where control beliefs are analysed in combination with social status and mortality risk during a six year observation period. Up to half of the mortality differences between status groups (in particular education) is 'explained' by control beliefs. When discussing the role of indirect selection in explaining these strong effects, the author suggests that 'socialized fatalism' in early life may determine educational and occupational attainment later in life and, thus, act as a confounder rather than a mediator. In both cases, however, options of intervention are justified that aim at strengthening the empowerment of less privileged socio-economic groups.

The inclusion of contextual factors, such as aggregate neighbourhood deprivation, into the analysis of social inequalities in health must be considered a major advance in this field. Frank J. van Lenthe provides an illuminating example of this progress. His chapter sets out to compare the size of the association between aggregate neighbourhood deprivation, as measured by the proportion of unemployed people in respective districts, and all-cause mortality across populations from six different countries: the Netherlands, the

United Kingdom, the United States, Finland, Italy and Spain. Using Cox proportional hazard models this association remained significant after adjusting for individual socio-economic status in most countries among men, but to a lesser extent among women. It is interesting to note that these results were obtained despite large variations in rates of country-specific aggregate deprivation. According to van Lenthe , this suggests that one or several common factors may underlie this association. Whether these factors concern social causation or social selection is not known, because most studies including the one discussed here are cross-sectional. Yet recent investigations suggest a dose-response relationship: the longer one lives in aggregate neighbourhood deprivation, the higher the risk of poor health. The chapter illustrates the promises as well as the limitations of current knowledge about contextual determinants of social variations in health and life expectancy.

The last two chapters further broaden the scope of analysis. Espen Dahl and colleagues start with the puzzling observation that the size of social inequalities in health in western Europe is about as large in more egalitarian countries as in more competitive, less egalitarian ones. In an attempt to tackle this problem, two lines of analysis are combined: comparative welfare state research and comparative health inequalities research. In its first part, the chapter deals with a discussion of current typologies of welfare state regimes, with special emphasis on the 'Nordic welfare state model'. This latter represents a rather homogeneous cluster with certain institutional features providing extended social benefits and services that favour social equality among citizens. Why should the Nordic welfare state model affect health inequalities? In the following parts of their chapter, authors propose several answers: social capital, decommodification, quality of work, and access to services including welfare state institutions for the elderly. When exploring the available evidence from comparative research on health inequalities, one cannot conclude that all Nordic countries under study document reduced relative and absolute inequalities in morbidity or mortality. This is mainly due to high social inequalities in Finland, where Nordic welfare policies were developed relatively recently. However, social inequalities in health are relatively smallest in these countries if income is chosen as an indicator. This may reflect a protective effect of reduced income inequality, but may also result from financial buffers against health-detrimental effects of economic recessions and shocks that are absent or less strong in neo-liberal welfare regimes.

As indicated in the title, this book is interested in new scientific evidence of health inequalities as well as its implications for policy. Although several individual chapters address this issue, the final chapter written by a leading expert in this field, Johan P. Mackenbach, deals with options of intervention in a systematic way. Starting with a discussion of national policy developments in western Europe that address health inequalities, the author concludes that Britain is now ahead of continental Europe in developing and implementing respective policies although important developments started in the Netherlands and Sweden. What type of evidence is needed to guide and support policies and interventions and is it acceptable to act on the basis of plausibility, given the often brief political 'windows of opportunity'? Ideally, according to Mackenbach, a three-step sequence should include (1) a theoretical rationale for intervention; (2) a theory-based intervention design, and (3) a demonstration of (cost)-effectiveness of this intervention. While such a general sequence is currently not available, promising intervention approaches evolving from prospective observational evidence are nevertheless justified, as far as their effectiveness is evaluated. In this regard, several results of the European Science Programme that are summarized in this volume offer new opportunities of health promotion, specifically among lower socio-economic groups. Examples include strengthening of coping resources among economically and psychosocially vulnerable groups of parents and children, health promotion programmes for schoolchildren, in combination with comprehensive policies that target socially deprived neighbourhood settings, and workplace health promotion strategies based on available theoretical concepts. Emphasis should be put on programmes that can be implemented on a sufficiently large scale to have an impact on population health.

Future directions

The contributions of this book extend the framework offered by the Black Report in several ways. First, they emphasize the importance of early life and socialization for adult health, and they test the refined concepts of latency, cumulation and pathways that offer a more adequate modelling of the impact of early life on unequal health later in life. Second, the chapters advance the case for robust associations between measures of an adverse psychosocial environment that is socially graded and ill health. This is demonstrated in two important areas of adult life, social relationships and work, where the role of cognitions and emotions and their psychobiological correlates are analysed in great detail. Finally, by taking macro-social contexts, such as aggregate neighbourhood deprivation, into account, the chapters broaden the scope of analysis as well as the frame of intervention policies.

Despite this progress research on social inequalities in health faces many more challenges, given the scope as well as the complexity of the problem.

Here, we only mention three challenges that, according to our view, deserve special attention in further advancing this important field of scientific inquiry.

The first challenge

The first challenge concerns social inequalities in health in older populations. Most investigations were interested in childhood, adolescence or midlife conditions, but rarely extended their scope of analysis into older age. It is true that the social gradient is steepest during midlife and decreases during the stages usually termed third and fourth age. Yet several reports document a continued social gradient of morbidity and mortality into old age in European populations (Marmot and Shipley 1996, van Rossum *et al.* 2000, Martelin 1994, Huisman *et al.* 2004). Although the relative inequalities between social groups decrease with age, it is likely that the absolute differences remain substantial, given the general increase of mortality in older age. To explain these differences, new approaches are needed. First, it will be important to define appropriate measures of socio-economic status for post-retirement populations. It was suggested that indicators of material resources, such as housing tenure or wealth, would matter more than previous occupational standing or educational attainment. In a different perspective, non-material aspects of social status, including prestige and access to privileged networks or sources of tangible support, may become more relevant. Second, the spectrum of health problems needs to be broadened. Inequalities in mental health and health functioning appear to widen in the post-retirement period. It is probable that this development coincides with an increased burden of cardiovascular and metabolic disorders that are more frequently clinically manifest among less privileged populations at this stage. In addition, disability and accidents in older age are socially graded.

A third approach concerns the extension of theoretical concepts from midlife to older life. Theoretical models, such as social support, high demand and low control, high effort and low reward, were mainly developed to explain social inequalities in health in midlife, with particular emphasis on work and employment and on family or community life. How important are they in explaining health differences later on? To what extent can they be adapted to the specific contexts of everyday life among the elderly? This question seems particularly relevant with regard to people entering the post-retirement stage of life where a mismatch has evolved between the strengths and capabilities of motivated people and a shortage of socially productive opportunities to realize their potential. Although people may be willing to put forth effort, there are generally not sufficient opportunities to act in new social roles past retirement and to experience personal need fulfilment and its beneficial health effects. It seems promising to further develop the notions of autonomy, control, reward and social reciprocity in view of these developments (Siegrist *et al.* 2004). On an epidemiological level, recent research demonstrates a link between productive activity and health among elderly people. For instance, in a prospective cohort study it was found that social and productive activities, such as volunteering or providing help to family and friends, were independently associated with length of overall survival (Glass *et al.* 1999). Again, the opportunity structure of social productivity past retirement is socially graded, and this fact may contribute to the unequal health burden of the elderly.

The second challenge

Population ageing is not restricted to modern Western societies, but affects large populations of rapidly developing countries, most visibly in Asia and in Latin America. This observation underscores the importance of a second challenge of future inequality research, the question of whether the explanatory approaches developed in Western industrialized societies can be successfully applied to societies with a different cultural background and different stages of the process of economic and societal modernization. It has been repeatedly stressed that modernization is rooted in European late medieval and early Renaissance developments which favoured the rise of modern capitalism, technological and scientific progress together with the transformation of political power. Starting with the industrial and political revolutions of the late eighteenth and early nineteenth century, the process of industrialization expanded beyond north-western Europe to include the United States and other regions of the world over the past 150 years.

This process was paralleled and, in part, influenced by specific cultural norms and attitudes stressing values such as personal achievement and individual autonomy or independence. In meritocratic societies, achieved social status to a considerable extent became contingent on personal performance, thus blaming those at the bottom of the societal structure (see the contribution of Bosma in Chapter 7). It may well be that the appraisal of social inequality, its meaning and significance varies according to cultural norms and attitudes. Moreover, it is not certain whether the theoretical concepts explaining the link between social inequality and health that were developed by scientists who were socialized into this Western culture, can be applied to observed social differences in health in societies with markedly different cultures and traditions.

Transcultural research that aims at explaining social inequalities in health is still in its infancy. However, first results from such studies are now available. They give some preliminary confirmation that the notions of control, support and reward at work are valid in different sociocultural contexts. For instance, the two work stress models described earlier have now been tested in several studies in Japan (Kawakami *et al.* 1998, Tsutsumi *et al.* 2001) and in China (Li *et al.* 2005, Xu *et al.* 2004). Their explanatory power is more than comparable to the one reported in Western studies, but cultural differences are visible as well. For instance, in a comparative study on conflict between work and home in Japan, Finland and Britain it was found that Japanese women had the greatest conflicts and poorest mental health while Finnish women had the lowest conflict and best mental health (Chandola *et al.* 2004). The former finding was interpreted in the context of powerful traditional gender attitudes to domestic labour in the Japanese culture.

In times of accelerated economic, technological and cultural globalization it will be important to investigate the generalizability of existing explanatory models of social inequalities in health and to draw respective conclusions for policy recommendations. Along these lines, the World Health Organization has recently established a Commission on Social Determinants of Health whose main task consists in transferring available scientific evidence to those regions of the world which have not yet created collective awareness of this problem and to influence decision-makers and stakeholders to change their policy agendas (Lee 2005, Marmot 2005). Moreover, the Commission aims to identifying successful interventions resulting in a reduction of health inequalities and to bring them to the attention of health policy organizations, both nationally and internationally.

The third challenge

Despite the fact that efforts to advance health among lower socio-economic population groups involve structural changes, the role of medicine and the medical profession as part of these efforts deserves careful consideration. Mainstream biomedical research is now moving towards genetic determinants of human diseases and their molecular mechanisms. Nevertheless, maintaining a dialogue between public health and biomedicine both at the theoretical and practical level, seems important and is considered a third challenge. With the availability of measures of genetic polymorphisms a new field of interdisciplinary research has evolved that is of potential interest to inequality research because it extends the notion of increased illness susceptibility in deprived people beyond the material and psychosocial dimensions to include genetic risk.

A prominent example of front line research may illustrate this argument. It is well known that the prevalence of critical life events is higher in lower social status groups and that their occurrence contributes to the onset of depressive disorders (Brown and Harris 1978). Yet depression is also more likely to become manifest in people whose genetic profile is characterized by two short alleles on a functional polymorphism of the serotonin transporter gene. Combining sociological information on critical life events with genetic information on alleles of the serotonin transporter gene increases the predictive power of incident depression above and beyond their additive value (Caspi *et al.* 2003). A practical result of these findings could consist in a more precise targeting of population groups at elevated risk which may improve the impact of preventive measures. Another example of potential benefit of integrating basic biomedical science into inequality research concerns advances in understanding shared pathophysiological pathways of different chronic diseases, such as cardiovascular diseases, metabolic disorders and depression. Chronic inflammation is one such shared mechanism. New immune markers including interleukin 6–gene polymorphisms may prove helpful in detecting early stages of illness susceptibility against which preventive activities can operate (Brunner 2002).

One of the key messages of this book is the importance of psychosocial factors associated with health inequalities and recent progress in their conceptualization and measurement. Negative social emotions such as anxiety, anger, frustration or disappointment are powerful stressors in the everyday lives of less privileged people. To understand the patterns of brain activation that occur when these emotions are experienced and how bodily stress mechanisms are elicited are important further steps of basic research. With the advent of available concepts and methods in brain research new opportunities of advancing our respective knowledge are given. Ideally, information on these processes will be linked to, and integrated with, epidemiological information on associations between exposure to an adverse psychosocial environment and incident disease.

A preliminary attempt towards this aim was undertaken in a recent experimental study where two groups of healthy men underwent functional magnetic resonance imaging while solving a series of mental arithmetic tasks. These tasks were either followed by monetary reward or omission of reward. The two groups were selected on the basis of high versus low scores measuring effort–reward imbalance at work. High scores reflect a history of chronic work-related reward frustration. In the group with high susceptibility to reward frustration, hyperactivation was observed in relevant parts of the brain reward system, the medial prefrontal, anterior cingulate and dorsolateral prefrontal cortex, during omission of an expected reward. The group with low susceptibility exhibited reduced activation, in line with prediction error theory. Findings may indicate a compromised ability of adapting brain activation among those suffering from chronic social reward frustration (Siegrist *et al.* 2005). However, we still do not have an adequate understanding of how the brain deals with the social world and how these negative emotions contribute to an increased burden of disease (Blakemore and Frith 2004).

These challenges, together with the findings and open questions presented in this book, document the promises and potential benefits of advanced research on social inequalities in health. It is our hope that improved interventions that aim at minimizing these inequalities will make appropriate use of this evidence.

References

Acheson D (1998). *Inequalities in health: Report of an independent inquiry.* HMSO, London.

Agency for Healthcare Research and Quality (2003). *National healthcare disparities report.* US Department of Health and Human Services, Rockville, MD.

Antonovsky A (1967). Social class life expectancy and overall mortality. *Milbank Memorial Fund Quarterly,* **45,** 31–73.

Arber S and Thomas H (2001). From women's health to a gender analysis of health. In: Cockerham WC, ed. *The Blackwell companion to medical sociology,* pp. 94–113. Blackwell, Oxford.

Berkman LF and Syme SL (1979). Social networks, host resistance and mortality: A nine- year follow-up of Alameda County residents. *American Journal of Epidemiology,* **109,** 186–204.

Blakemore SJ and Frith U (2004). How does the brain deal with the social world? *NeuroReport,* **15,** 119–28.

Bourdieu P (1993). *The field of cultural production.* Columbia University Press, New York.

Brown GW and Harris TO (1978). *Social origins of depression.* Tavistock, London.

Brunner E (2002). Stress mechanisms in coronary heart disease. In: Stansfeld SA and Marmot MG, eds. *Stress and the heart,* pp. 181–99. BMJ Books, London.

Caspi A, Sugden K, Moffitt TE *et al.* (2003). Influence of life stress on depression. .Moderation by a polymorphism in the 5-HTT-gene. *Science,* **301,** 386–9.

Chandola T, Martikainen P, Bartley M *et al.* (2004). Does conflict between home and work explain the effect of multiple roles on mental health? A comparative study of Finland, Japan, and the UK. *International Journal of Epidemiology,* **33,** 884–93.

Daniels N (1996). Justice, fair procedures, and the goals of medicine. *Hastings Center Reports,* **26,** 10–22.

Davey Smith G, Bartley M and Blane D (1990). The Black Report on socioeconomic inequalities in health 10 years on. *British Medical Journal,* **301,** 373–7.

Diez-Roux A (1998). Bringing context back to epidemiology: variables and fallacies in multilevel analysis. *American Journal of Public Health,* **88,** 216–22.

Drever F and Whitehead M (eds) (1997). *Health inequalities.* The Stationery Office, London.

Elstad JI (2000). *Social inequalities in health and their explanations.* Rapport 9/00. NOVA, Oslo.

Fox J (ed.) (1989). *Health inequalities in European countries.* Gower, Aldershot.

Glass TA, Mendes de Leon C, Marottuli RA and Berkman LF (1999). Population-based study of social productive activities as predictors of survival among elderly Americans. *British Medical Journal*, **319**, 478–83.

Gubéran E and Usel M (2000). *Mortalité prématurée et invalidité selon la profession et la classe sociale à Genève*. Final report. OCIRT, Geneva.

Huisman H, Kunst AE, Andersen O *et al.* (2004). Socioeconomic inequalities in mortality among elderly people in 11 European populations. *Journal of Epidemiology and Community Health*, **58**, 468–75.

Kadushin C (1964). Social class and the experience of ill health. *Sociological Inquiry*, **534**, 67–80.

Karasek R and Theorell T (1990). *Healthy work: stress, productivity, and the reconstruction of working life*. Basic Books, New York.

Kawakami N, Haratani T and Araki S (1998). Job strain and arterial blood pressure, serum cholesterol, and smoking as risk factors for coronary heart disease in Japan. *International Archives of Occupational and Environmental Health*, **71**, 429–32.

Kitagawa EM and Hauser PM (1973). *Differential mortality in the United States: a study in socio-economic epidemiology*. Harvard University Press, Cambridge, MA.

Krieger N (2005). Defining and investigating social disparities in cancer: critical issues. *Cancer Causes and Control*, **16**, 5–14.

Krieger N, Williams DR and Moss NE (1997). Measuring social class in US public health research: concepts, methodologies, and guidelines. *Annual Review of Public Health*, **18**, 341–78.

Kuh D, Ben-Shlomo Y (eds) (2004). *A life course approach to chronic disease epidemiology*. Oxford University Press, Oxford.

Kunst AE (1997). *Cross-national comparisons of socio-economic differences in mortality*. Ph.D. Thesis, Erasmus University, Rotterdam.

Lahelma E (2001). Health and social stratification. In WC Cockerham, ed. *The Blackwell companion to medical sociology*, pp. 64–93. Blackwell Publishers, Oxford.

Lee JW (2005). Public health is a social issue. *Lancet*, **365**, 1005–6.

Li J, Wenjie Y, Cheng Y, Siegrist J and Cho S-I (2005). Effort–reward imbalance at work and job dissatisfaction in Chinese healthcare workers: a validation study. *International Archives of Occupational and Environmental Health*, **78**, 198–204.

Lynch JW, Davey-Smith G, Kaplan GA and House JS (2000). Income inequality and mortality: importance to health of individual income, psychosocial environment, or material conditions. *British Medical Journal*, **320**, 1200–4.

Macintyre S (1997). The Black report and beyond: what are the issues? *Social Science and Medicine*, **44**, 723–45.

Mackenbach JP (2005). Community genetics or public health genetics? *Journal of Epidemiology and Community Health*, **59**, 179–80.

Mackenbach JP and Bakker M (eds) (2002. *Reducing inequalities in health. A European perspective*. Routledge, London.

Mackenbach JP, Kunst AE, Cavelaars AD, Groenhof F and Geurts JJ (1997). Socioeconomic inequalities in morbidity and mortality in Western Europe. The EU working group on socioeconomic inequalities in health. *Lancet*, **349**, 1655–9.

Marmot M (2004). *Status syndrome: How your social standing directly affects your health and life expectancy.* Bloomsbury, London.

Marmot M (2005). Social determinants of health inequalities. *The Lancet*, **365**, 1099–104.

Marmot M and Shipley MJ (1996). Do socio-economic differences in mortality persist after retirement? 25-year follow-up of civil servants from the first Whitehall Study. *British Medical Journal*, **313**, 1177–80.

Marmot MG and McDowall ME (1986). Mortality decline and widening social inequalities. *Lancet*, **2**, 274–6.

Marmot MG and Siegrist J (eds) (2004). Health inequalities and the psychosocial environment. Special Issue: *Social Science and Medicine*, **58**, 1461–574.

Marmot MG and Wilkinson RG (2001). Psychosocial and material pathways in the relation between income and health: a response to Lynch et al. *British Medical Journal*, **322**, 1233–6.

Marmot MG and Wilkinson RG (eds) (2006). *Social determinants of health, 2nd edn.* Oxford University Press, Oxford.

Marmot MG, Adelstein AM, Robinson N and Rose G. (1978). The changing social class distribution of heart disease. *British Medical Journal*, **ii**, 1109–12.

Marmot MG, Davey Smith G, Stansfeld S *et al.* (1991). Health inequalities among British civil servants: The Whitehall II study. *Lancet*, **337**, 387–93.

Marmot MG, Shipley MJ and Rose G (1984). Inequalities in death-specific explanations of a general pattern. *Lancet*, **i**, 1003–6.

Martelin T (1994). Mortality by indicators of socioeconomic status among the Finnish elderly. *Social Science and Medicine*, **38**, 1257–78.

McEwen BS (1998). Protective and damaging effects of stress mediators. *New England Journal of Medicine*, **338**, 171–9.

Nettle D (2003). Intelligence and class mobility in the British population. *British Journal of Psychology*, **94**, 551–61.

Pappas G, Queen S, Hadden W and Fisher G (1993). The increasing disparity in mortality between socio-economic groups in the United States, 1960 and 1986. *New England Journal of Medicine*, **329**, 103–9.

Rawls J (2001. *Justice as fairness.* Harvard University Press, Boston, MA.

Sacker A, Firth D, Fitzpatrick R, Lynch K and Bartley M (2000). Comparing health inequality in men and women: prospective study of mortality, 1986–1996. *British Medical Journal*, **320**, 1303–7.

Siegrist J (1996). Adverse health effects of high effort–low reward conditions at work. *Journal of Occupational Health Psychology*, **1**, 27–43.

Siegrist J and Marmot M (2004). Health inequalities and the psychosocial environment – two scientific challenges. *Social Science and Medicine*, **58**, 1463–73.

Siegrist J and Weyers S (2004). *ESF Programme Social Variations in Health Expectancy in Europe.* Available at http://uni-duesseldorf.de/health.

Siegrist J, Knesebeck OvD and Pollack CE (2004). Social productivity and well-being of older people: a sociological exploration. *Social Theory and Health*, **1**, 1–17.

Siegrist J, Menrath I, Stoecker T, Klein M, Kellermann T, Shah J, Zilles K, Schneider F (2005). Differential brain activation according to chronic social reward frustration. *NeuroReport*, **16**, 1899–903.

Singh-Manoux A and Marmot M (2005). The role of socialisation in explaining social inequalities in health. *Social Science and Medicine*, **60**, 2129–33.

Townsend P and Davidson N (eds) (1982). *Inequalities in health: The Black Report and the health divide*. Penguin Books, Harmondsworth.

Tsutsumi A, Kayaba K, Theorell T and Siegrist J (2001) Association between job stress and depression among Japanese employees threatened by job loss in a comparison between two complementary job-stress models. *Scandinavian Journal of Work, Environment and Health*, **27**, 146–53.

Valkonen T, Sihvonen AP and Lahelma E (1997). Health expectancy by level of education in Finland. *Social Science and Medicine*, **44**, 801–8.

Van Rossum CTM, Shipley MJ, Van de Mheen H, Grobbee DE and Marmot MG (2000). Employment grade differences in cause specific mortality. A 25-year follow-up of civil servants from the first Whitehall study. *Journal of Epidemiology and Community Health*, **54**, 178–84.

Williams RB (1998). Lower socioeconomic status and increased mortality: early childhood roots and the potential for successful interventions. *The Journal of the American Medical Association*, **279**, 1745–6.

Xu L, Siegrist J, Cao W, Li L, Tomlinson B and Chan J (2004). Measuring job stress and family stress in Chinese working women: a validation study focusing on blood pressure and psychosomatic symptoms. *Women and Health*, **39**, 31–46.

Chapter 2

Life course development of unequal health

Chris Power and Diana Kuh

Introduction

Risk of death is socially graded, with individuals from the least socio-economically advantaged groups having the highest mortality rates and those in the most advantaged positions having the lowest rates. The extent of social inequality in health throughout Europe was demonstrated in a comparative study of mortality in manual and non-manual social classes for men in 11 countries from the northern and southern part of western Europe. Inequalities in mortality from all causes were found in all countries, although varying in magnitude: among 45–59 year old men the rate ratio ranged from 1.71 (95 per cent CI 1.66, 1.77) in Finland to 1.33 (1.30, 1.36) in Denmark (Kunst *et al.* 1998, Mackenbach *et al.* 1997). Despite the difficulties of making comparisons across countries that arise from differences in the way that data are collected and classified, the evidence suggests that higher occupational groups are better able to avoid premature death.

That social inequalities in health exist is not in doubt, but the causes of inequality, despite being an important focus of research (Fox 1989), are not well understood. In recent decades, there has been growing evidence that exposures across different stages of life affect adult health outcomes, and a life course approach has now been applied to research on social inequalities in health (Davey Smith and Lynch 2004, Power and Matthews 1997, Power *et al.* 1998, van de Mheen *et al.* 1998). A life course approach investigates how *social* and *biological* factors operating at different stages of the life course and across generations contribute to the development of inequalities in adult health and disease. In particular, it asks how much of the inequality in adult health is due to socially patterned environmental exposures in early life, acting through 'developmental health', such as physical growth, emotional and cognitive development, or through health behaviours and social pathways.In this chapter we illustrate some of the key findings emerging from this new literature that examines how factors acting at different life stages might contribute towards the development of unequal health. In doing so, we draw heavily on our work based on the Medical Research Council National Survey of Health and Development (NSHD) and the National Child Development Study (NCDS), otherwise known as the 1946 and 1958 British birth cohort studies (Ferri *et al.* 2003). We mention emerging conceptual frameworks, terminology and methodological challenges in life course epidemiology only briefly as these have been dealt with more fully elsewhere (Ben-Shlomo and Kuh 2002, Graham and Power 2004, Kuh *et al.* 2003).

Our central focus in this chapter is with the question: Do exposures earlier in life influence the development of inequalities in adult health outcomes? An additional question is: How much of the adult socio-economic gradient is explained by factors occurring earlier on? In addressing these questions we first identify factors from early and later life stages that are implicated in the development of adult disease and show that many of these factors are socially patterned. Second, we report on effects of the socio-economic environment in early life on adult inequalities in mortality, morbidity and health behaviour, using a simple approach that tests whether any effects act through or independently of the adult socio-economic environment. Third, we discuss why it is important, from a life course perspective on the development of unequal health, to consider health and functional trajectories as well as the more conventional outcomes of morbidity and mortality. We present a conceptual framework that outlines the ways in which the early socio-economic environment can affect the development of inequalities in adult health, and then provide examples that illustrate these pathways in relation to a diverse range of adult outcomes. These include psychological distress, coronary heart disease (CHD), lung function and physical capability.

Factors from early and later life increase the risk of adult disease

Risk factors for two common adult health problems, CHD and respiratory disease, illustrate the extent to which disease status is affected by exposures spanning the entire life course. For CHD, and starting with the earliest life stages, disease risk has been shown (Davey Smith *et al.* 2001, Lawlor *et al.* 2004) to increase in association with:

- poor growth *in utero* and also postnatally, as indicated with measures of fetal growth, namely lower birthweight, shorter leg length and height, but also with measures of accelerated postnatal growth, particularly weight gain;
- poor *lifetime* socio-economic conditions: adversity in early life is a major influence on early growth patterns and as mentioned later in the chapter

there are now many studies showing that socio-economic factors both early on and later influence CHD risk;

+ abdominal obesity;

+ dietary fat;

+ binge drinking;

+ factors unique to women (possibly including later age of menarche, higher parity, early menopause and exogenous oestrogen, although for some of these factors evidence to date is limited and inconsistent and effects may be due, in some instances, to other socio-economic and behavioural factors) (Lawlor *et al.* 2002);

+ diabetes and insulin resistance syndrome;

+ classical adult risk factors (smoking, hypertension, cholesterol, obesity, physical inactivity).

In addition many of these adult risk factors, such as diabetes, obesity, hypertension and early menopause, have been shown to be influenced by factors operating in early life (Kuh and Ben-Shlomo 2004).

For respiratory disease several factors are implicated, though there is debate and controversy about the magnitude and direction of effects for some of them (Strachan and Sheikh 2004). Also, relationships may be changing as respiratory illness due to asthma and allergy becomes more common. Adult respiratory disease is increased for those with:

+ poor growth *in utero*;

+ early infection and chest illness;

+ poor postnatal growth and short height;

+ passive smoking in early life;

+ larger family size, overcrowded homes and poorer socio-economic circumstances. (A different pattern is emerging for asthma and allergy where the risk is seen for smaller families and higher rather than lower social class);

+ diet, notably fresh fruit and vegetables, with some studies suggesting that forced expiratory volume in one second (FEV1) is lower among individuals with lower consumption of fresh fruit;

+ pollution: 'old' (smoke, sulphur dioxide) and 'new' (e.g. related to vehicle emissions) pollutants;

+ classical risk factors (smoking – passive and own behaviour – occupational exposures).

Some influences associated with socio-economic circumstances, such as smoking – both own and passive – as well as possibly pollution, are likely to be acting across the life course to affect respiratory illness later in adulthood.

There are many other adult diseases for which known risk factors include those that are current or recent influences and others that originate earlier in life (Kuh and Ben-Shlomo 2004, Kuh and Hardy 2002), including breast cancer, musculoskeletal disorders, depression and neuropsychiatric outcomes.

Social patterning of risk factors at different life stages

In order to gain a better understanding of the development of health inequalities we need evidence that factors at different life stages are not only related to adult disease outcomes but are also socially patterned. Such evidence would suggest that these influences contribute to the development of health inequalities in adult life. Many risk factors are socially patterned: poorer growth *in utero*, postnatal weight gain, household overcrowding and larger family size all decrease in prevalence from groups with unskilled manual social backgrounds to those with professional and managerial social backgrounds (Power and Matthews 1997).

To illustrate, childhood height tends to be lower in less advantaged social groups: in the 1958 British birth cohort, children with fathers in unskilled manual occupations were shorter at age 7, by about 3 cm, than those from professional and managerial households (Power and Matthews 1997), suggesting that growth is impaired or delayed by adverse socio-economic circumstances. Compensatory growth often follows adversity in early life, but growth deficits can be long-lasting, as seen in persisting height deficits through to adulthood of those in the 1958 cohort from poorer socio-economic backgrounds (Li *et al.* 2004).

A second example for which we have evidence of social patterning of risk at early life stages is exposure to tobacco. Within the 1958 cohort, those born into unskilled manual backgrounds (social classes IV and V) were more likely to have been exposed to tobacco *in utero* than those with professional and managerial backgrounds (classes I and II) and they were more likely to live in homes where a parent smoked when they were aged 16. Among males, for example, the social difference was 47 per cent vs. 30 per cent for exposure *in utero* and 79 per cent vs. 48 per cent at age 16 (Power and Matthews 1997). During young adulthood, those with unskilled manual backgrounds at birth were also more likely to be regular smokers. These observations are well-known, but it is worth emphasizing that the social pattern of exposure started very early in life, continued throughout childhood and into early adulthood, well before many health consequences are experienced. Social gradients in smoking among the female cohort members were occurring during their own reproductive years, thereby demonstrating differential social transmission of risk to the next generation.

Contribution of early and later life to unequal health: a simple approach

Before considering how *specific* exposures from different life stages affect adult health inequalities, we should not overlook a simple general approach that has yielded valuable clues on the timing of risk exposures. A growing number of studies have investigated the importance of influences at different life stages for adult health inequalities by comparing effects of child and adult socio-economic position (SEP). One example of a comparison of mortality is available from the 1946 British birth cohort (Kuh *et al.* 2002b). By age 54, those from manual origins (i.e. with a father in a manual job during their early childhood, when they were age four) were twice as likely to have died in adult life than those from non-manual origins (6 vs. 3 per cent). The rate was almost double across all ages at which adult mortality was studied (26 to 54 years). Deaths over this age range were also influenced by adult SEP, with an unadjusted hazard ratio for manual versus non-manual occupation at age 26 of 1.6. Whilst the hazard ratio associated with adult social class reduced to 1.4 after adjustment for childhood social class, the hazard ratio of about 2 observed for childhood was little affected by allowing for class in early adulthood. This demonstrates that the influence of childhood social class on mortality is not just a reflection of adult social class effects: both child and adult socio-economic position therefore appear to influence mortality risk. Combining information on child and adult social class showed even bigger effects on mortality, with an almost threefold risk of premature death for those in a manual class on both occasions. Using another adult socio-economic indicator (housing tenure) the risk for those not owning their own homes and coming from manual origins in relation to those who owned their homes and came from non manual origins was almost fivefold (Kuh *et al.* 2002b).

Such studies provide a powerful demonstration of influences from childhood acting on adult mortality. We would, however, expect considerable variation in relationships for different causes of death to underlie this general pattern for all-cause mortality. This is illustrated in the findings from the West of Scotland Collaborative Study, a cohort of 5766 men aged 35–64 at baseline with retrospective data on childhood SEP. Before adjustment for adult SEP excess risks of dying from CHD, lung cancer, respiratory disease, stroke and stomach cancer were observed for men from manual compared with non-manual social origins. Different patterns emerged after adjusting for adult SEP and risk factors (Davey Smith *et al.* 1998). For lung cancer, the excess risk associated with manual social origins virtually disappeared after adjustment, from an age-adjusted relative death rate of 1.65 (95 per cent CI 1.12, 2.43) to 1.23 (0.81, 1.88) after further adjustment for adult social position (occupational class, deprivation category and car use). This reduction suggests that the most important risk factors for lung cancer, almost certainly smoking in this case, operate in adult life. For CHD and respiratory disease the excess risk of death was considerably attenuated after adjustment, with relative rates reducing from 1.52 (1.24, 1.87) to 1.28 (1.03, 1.61) for CHD; and from 2.01 (1.17, 3.48) to 1.53 (0.85, 2.75) for respiratory disease. Hence, for CHD and respiratory disease, factors operating across the life course, in both childhood and adult life, appear to affect adult outcome. For stroke and stomach cancer, the excess risk associated with the childhood social environment (1.83 and 2.06 respectively) hardly changed, implicating factors that operate in early life in the aetiology of these diseases. For stomach cancer we now know that this is likely to be exposure to *helicobacter pylori*. For stroke, evidence is scant although research in cohort and ecological studies suggests that childhood social conditions are possibly more relevant for haemorrhagic as compared with ischaemic stroke, with long-term effects of early infectious disease as a potential explanation for this association (Galobardes *et al*. 2004). Lifetime socio-economic circumstances have also been shown to be important for measures of morbidity, as well as for mortality. In the 1958 cohort, both childhood and adult SEP were associated with the study participant's rating of their health at age 33 (Power *et al*. 1999). Using a lifetime socio-economic score based on social class at four time points (birth and ages 16, 23, 33 years), there were striking differences in the proportions rating their health as poor or fair, ranging from about 5 per cent of men and women in the most favourable lifetime circumstances to 20–25 per cent of those in the least favourable circumstances.

Other measures relevant to adult health have been investigated in this way. For example, effects of childhood SEP on both quitting smoking and obesity are seen across several studies in Europe and the US (Figure 2.1) (Power *et al*. 2005). These findings are of interest because they demonstrate an influence of childhood SEP on obesity risk that is not merely reflecting adult circumstances: both child and adult SEP affect an important determinant of adult health. Further work examining possible explanations for the childhood SEP effect has suggested that it is not explained by birth weight or childhood weight status, as shown in relation to the trajectory of body mass index (BMI) from age 20–43 years in the 1946 cohort (Hardy *et al*. 2000); and it is also independent of educational qualifications, as shown for obesity at 33 years in the 1958 cohort (Power *et al*. 2003). We will return to this issue later in the chapter, as the associations with childhood SEP are relevant to inequalities in cardiovascular disease in adulthood.

For smoking, we would expect that adult trends are predominantly influenced by SEP in adulthood, an expectation that is confirmed in our comparison of SEP effects across several study populations (Power *et al.* 2005). Nonetheless, Figure 2.1 provides some evidence that childhood SEP also matters, in particular to quitting behaviour, especially for women. The higher levels of cigarette consumption (and therefore nicotine dependence) known to be associated with a manual social class background offer one possible explanation for the influence of childhood SEP on adult smoking. Interestingly, levels of consumption did not account for the childhood SEP effect on adult smoking in the 1958 cohort (Jefferis *et al.* 2003), suggesting that other processes are operating through which childhood SEP affects smoking, at least in relation to quitting smoking.

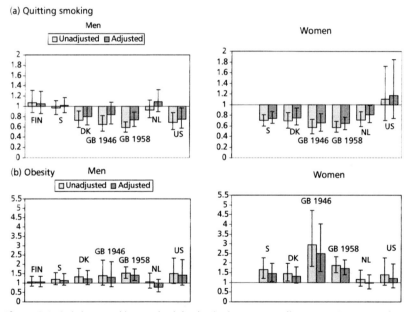

Figure 2.1 Quitting smoking and adult obesity in seven studies across Europe and the US: association (Odds Ratio and 95 per cent confidence interval) with childhood manual socio-economic position.*

*Age-adjusted ORs and adjusted for adult SEP: non-manual is the reference category.

Obesity (BMI ≥ 30 kg/m²).

Country abbreviations: FIN = Finland, S = Sweden, DK = Denmark, GB 1946 = 1946 British birth cohort, GB 1958 = 1958 British birth cohort, NL = Netherlands, US = United States.

Source: Power *et al.* 2005.

Trajectories of health and functional status

There are several reasons why studies on the life course development of unequal health should look at function as well as disease status and health behaviour. One reason is that social and physical environments may leave imprints on the structure or function of body systems (Barker 1998). Moreover, function is a way of looking at health across the life course, which can interact with social factors over time. Hence, functional trajectories provide a more dynamic concept than a mortality/disease categorization, incorporating the natural history and physiological trajectory of biological systems. Many functions display rapid growth and development in the early stages of life, followed by a period of stability or plateau and a gradual decline with age. This is illustrated in Figure 2.2 for lung function (Strachan and Sheikh 2004), but the pattern also applies to cognitive function, muscle function and so forth. Periods of rapid development may occur during a limited time window or 'critical period' during which exposures can have adverse or protective effects on development and subsequent disease outcome. Outside this developmental window there is no excess disease risk associated with exposure (Kuh *et al.* 2003). Environmental factors in early life may influence either the development of capital or reserve ('gain' in Figure 2.2) or the rate of decline ('loss' in Figure 2.2), whereas factors acting later in life can only affect the rate of decline. Many functional measures are outcomes in their own right (for example, lung, muscle and cognitive function) and are risk factors for later disease. We therefore need to look at function across the life course.

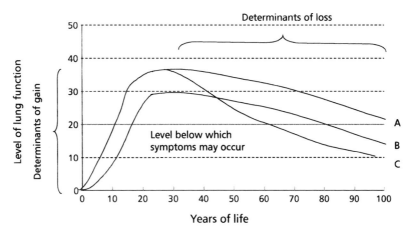

Figure 2.2 Lung function across the life course. Modified from Strachan and Sheikh (2004).

A = normal development and decline; B = exposure in early life reducing lung function potential; C = exposure acting in mid-life accelerating age-related decline.

Studies of functional trajectories have the potential to clarify the pathways through which factors operating at different life stages lead eventually to increased disease risk. One focus of such studies might be to look at socio-economic differences in how function is acquired and lost. This involves some assessment of health capital and of health potential. By *health capital* we mean the accumulation of biological resources, inherited or acquired during earlier stages of life that shape current function and health status. We include resilience to future environmental insults as part of health capital, a term which we regard as analogous to the idea of constitution used in the inter-war years. By *health potential* we mean the chance of survival and optimal functioning and of maintaining and improving positive health attributes and discarding or reducing negative ones.

For those at the beginning of life studies of functional status might focus on the differential chances for full physical and mental development, whilst for older persons, an assessment of the differential chances of delaying degenerative ageing processes would be of central importance. Life course studies allow us to assess, for example, how level of functioning at one age affects the level of functioning (impairment) or disease at another. With measures that at least discriminate across the mild end of dysfunction and ideally discriminate those at the higher end of functioning, it may be possible to establish whether there are threshold effects or whether improved level of functioning across the whole range is always more optimal for current health and future health potential. Later in the chapter we will discuss life course relationships for selected examples of functional measures.

Conceptual life course frameworks linking childhood socio-economic environment to adult health

There are clearly many ways in which the early socio-economic environment can affect health many years later and these life course relationships are presented in a conceptual framework in Figure 2.3. As with other similar conceptual frameworks (Kuh *et al.* 2004a), Figure 2.3 is a simplification of interacting social and biological processes commencing early in life. The framework is described in greater detail elsewhere (Graham and Power 2004), but several points are noteworthy here. First, it puts childhood disadvantage as stemming from the mother and her partner, starting from before birth and throughout childhood (large grey box), and thereby representing the enduring context in which the child is conceived, born and grows up. Four pathways are set in this context, including the development of (1) physical and emotional health, (2) health behaviours, (3) cognitive development and educational progress, and (4) social identities, such as those associated with early parenthood. These four dimensions are identified in the framework as central to the link between childhood disadvantage and poor adult health.

The concept of 'developmental health' is captured by the framework. This is a broad rather than narrow concept of health in childhood, embracing cognitive, social and emotional development as well as physical development because of their importance for adult outcomes, including health status (Keating and Hertzman 1999). Figure 2.3 includes this range of developmental trajectories, and indicates the different ways in which these dimensions of development may operate to influence adult health. Physical and emotional health and health behaviour in childhood are seen as acting primarily as direct effects on health and functional status in adulthood, whereas the influence of cognitive development and educational performance, together with the identities through which young people negotiate their transition to adulthood, are seen primarily as more indirect pathways: these dimensions are represented as shaping socio-economic circumstances in adulthood, circumstances which in turn have a major influence on adult health. Figure 2.3 recognizes that socio-economic factors at different life stages may operate either via *social chains of risk* or by influencing exposures to causal factors at earlier life stages which form part of long-term *biological or psychological chains of risk*. The conceptual framework accommodates processes involving critical periods, cumulative and chains of risk, which though theoretically distinct processes are *not* necessarily mutually exclusive (Kuh *et al.* 2003).

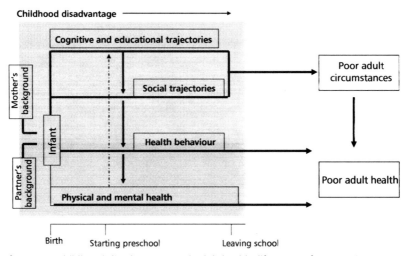

Figure 2.3 Childhood disadvantage and adult health: life-course framework.
Source: Graham and Power 2004.

Building more complex life course models to study the development of unequal health

While comparisons of effects of SEP at different life stages have yielded important clues on the timing of influences affecting the development of unequal health in adulthood, it is clear from the conceptual framework presented in Figure 2.3 that more complex models are needed if we are to understand the processes involved. Some recent research attempts to build more comprehensive life course analyses of unequal health and our purpose in this section is to illustrate some of the work in this area with selected examples on psychological distress, CHD, lung function and physical capability.

The unequal development of psychological distress and self-rated poor health

Life course influences on a range of psychological disorders, such as depression, have long been recognized, with several early life factors implicated as well as adult factors (Brown and Harris 1978, Maughan and McCarthy 1997, Robins 1978), including, for example:

- insecure attachment in early life, and influences impeding the attachment process;
- early adversity (such as parental conflict or separation and their poor mental health, being raised in an institution, i.e., being 'in care');
- adolescent behaviour;
- lone/teenage parenthood;
- lacking emotional support, such as confiding relationships;
- work stress, including job insecurity and adverse working conditions;
- family stress, including conflict in relationships and separation.

These are only some of the factors identified from the literature but they nonetheless indicate the extent to which the entire life span, starting with the very earliest months of infancy, may be involved in the development of some adult psychological disorders. In the context of the development of unequal adult health, it is notable that many influences are socially patterned. For example, within the 1958 birth cohort, both parental separation/divorce and teenage pregnancy increased in frequency from those with professional/ managerial background to those with unskilled manual backgrounds: among women, the percentages for parental separation were 14 to 24 respectively; for teenage pregnancy they were 4 to 18. Other relevant factors show similarly graded patterns (Power and Matthews 1997).

In further work on the 1958 cohort, analyses focused on our central question, namely, do early life factors contribute to the development of inequalities in adult outcome? For the purposes of this work we used a generic measure, psychological 'distress' (the Malaise Inventory), as an available outcome rather than measures for specific disorders (Power *et al.* 2002). Figure 2.4 shows odds ratios (OR) for psychological distress at age 33, as the adult health outcome used in this study: both men and women in unskilled manual classes had a more than threefold risk of psychological distress relative to professional and managerial classes. The OR associated with social class representing health inequality, reduced to about two when allowance was made for factors occurring during childhood, from birth to adolescence, suggesting that childhood factors were contributing to the class differential. The main childhood factors accounting for the class difference (OR), which may in part be markers of early distress, were:

- cognitive ability, assessed by teachers when the study participant was aged seven, accounting for reductions of 26 per cent (males) and 23 per cent (females);
- socio-emotional adjustment between ages 7 and 16, accounting for reductions of 19 per cent (males) and 13 per cent (females);
- physical development, as represented by height at age seven, accounting for reductions of 1 per cent (males) and 5 per cent (females).

Although the reductions in OR reported above are from analyses that did not adjust for other factors, they indicate nonetheless that cognition and socio-emotional adjustment in childhood, and thereby the factors that have an influence on them, contribute to the development of social inequalities in psychological distress in adulthood. But even with allowance for several childhood factors, Figure 2.4 suggests there is still substantial inequality in psychological distress that remains to be explained. Adult life factors also contribute to the development of unequal psychological distress: the class differential is virtually abolished with further adjustment for factors in adult life, particularly early child-bearing and financial hardship for women, and work factors – job strain and insecurity – for men. These findings suggest that gradients for psychological distress reflect the cumulative effect of multiple adversities experienced from childhood (Power *et al.* 2002).

Another adult health outcome that we have investigated in the 1958 cohort is poor rated health, which is now recognized as an indicator of later ill-health and mortality (Idler and Benyamini 1997). For poor/fair rated health at age 33, the odds in classes IV and V (relative to I and II) are

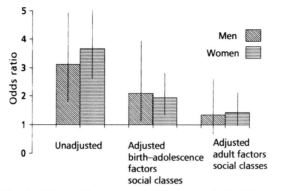

Figure 2.4 Odd ratios (IV and V versus I and II) for psychological distress: 1958 birth cohort at age 33.

Source: Power *et al.* 2002.

Psychological 'distress' is a generic measure, based on the Malaise Inventory, rather than a measure indicating a specific disorder.

[†] Birth to adolescence factors include: social class at birth, ability (five skills) at age seven years, housing tenure at age 11 years, parental aspirations for and interest in their child's education, behaviour ages 7 to 16 years, institutional care, school qualifications.

[#] Adult factors include: age at first child, unemployment, financial hardship, psychosocial work strain, job insecurity.

3.15 (95 per cent CI 2.04, 4.88) for men and 2.30 (1.34, 3.94) for women (Power *et al.* 1998). After adjustment for factors from birth to adolescence (early socio-economic circumstances, behaviour, smoking, school qualifications) the reduction in the OR is substantial: to 2 for men and 1.5 for women. With adjustment for factors in adult life (smoking, adult socio-economic circumstances, job insecurity, age at first child) the social class differential is abolished. For this health indicator the conclusion is similar to that for psychological distress, in that inequalities are not due to a single cause, but are more likely to develop as a result of exposures starting early in life and across childhood, through to more recent influences in adulthood.

Contribution of childhood growth and lifetime weight gain to the unequal development of coronary heart disease

Findings from the Whitehall II study and other cohort studies have been instrumental in focusing attention on socio-economic differentials in CHD (see Chapter 1). Marmot and his colleagues reported an association between short height and CHD twenty years ago, findings suggestive of an effect of early life influences (Marmot *et al.* 1984). Barker has emphasized the potential relevance of the intrauterine and early postnatal environment in explanations for social inequalities in CHD (Barker 1991). Davey Smith and his colleagues have been the most systematic in assessing the role of risk factors acting in childhood and across the whole life course as explanations for adult socio-economic differentials in CHD (Davey Smith *et al.* 2001). In a recent review (Davey Smith and Lynch 2004), 24 studies were identified that have investigated the relationship between childhood socio-economic circumstances and CHD. The evidence indicates a small but consistent effect of adverse childhood socio-economic circumstances on CHD, independent of later life circumstances. The 15 prospective studies generally show a stronger effect of childhood circumstances. Studies that have been able to adjust for adult behavioural factors like smoking or proximal risk factors suggest these factors explain some but by no means all of the relationship.

An alternative possibility is that the relationship between poor childhood socio-economic circumstances and adult CHD may be explained by prenatal or postnatal growth. Few studies have both measures of growth and early socio-economic position, and those that do rarely address this question. An exception was the US Nurses' Health study, which showed no attenuation of the relationship between coming from blue collar family of origin and adult CHD in 117,000 women, after adjusting for birthweight, breastfeeding and adult height (Gliksman *et al.* 1995). This study was limited by its retrospective measures. Another study (Eriksson *et al.* 2001) was carried out by Barker and colleagues, based on a cohort of 3,676 men born in Helsinki between 1933–44 where measures of size at birth, childhood height and weight, and markers of childhood SEP were collected prospectively. Their analysis focused on an interaction between early growth and adult circumstances, showing that adverse effects on hospitalization or death from CHD of low ponderal index at birth and accelerated weight gain between 1 and 12 years were stronger in men who ended up in poor adult socio-economic circumstances. Father's socio-economic circumstances were seen to be less important than these other factors. A second study (Eriksson *et al.* 2004) on hypertension in 6730 men and women from the same cohort, restored the importance of childhood circumstances by showing that the effects of birthweight, ponderal index and accelerated weight gain were stronger for those whose fathers had been labourers than those with fathers from the middle class.

Figure 2.5 shows how the difference in hospitalization or death from CHD by father's social class was affected by adjustment for childhood growth and later SEP in the Helsinki cohort (C Osmond, unpublished). The unadjusted hazard ratio shows that men whose fathers were labourers compared with

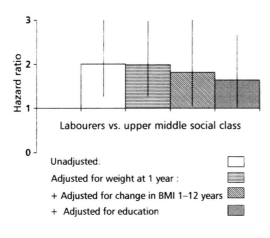

Figure 2.5 Hazard ratios (95 per cent confidence intervals) for CHD in men by childhood socio-economic position (labourers vs. upper middle social class). Helsinki 1933–44 cohort. Clive Osmond, personal communication.

men whose fathers were from the upper middle class had double the risk of CHD. The first adjustment shows that there was no effect on the social differential after allowing for infant weight at age one year. The second adjustment, for change in childhood BMI, attenuates the effect of childhood circumstances somewhat more, as does the final adjustment for the level of education (Figure 2.5). There was no information on adult BMI in this Helsinki cohort so we cannot test whether the effect of weight gain after age 12 explains more of the childhood social class effect on CHD.

Further insight into the role of early growth in the development of inequalities in CHD risk can be gleaned from findings from the 1946 British birth cohort comparing the childhood social class and birthweight effects on the change in adult blood pressure, measured at 36, 43 and 53 years (Hardy *et al.* 2003). The regression coefficients for separate models fitted at each age and adjusted for sex indicated that lower birthweight and coming from manual origins were associated with a higher systolic blood pressure at all three ages. Using multi-level models with blood pressure as a repeated outcome and the intercept based on blood pressure values at age 36 years, there was a significant and consistent effect of birthweight on blood pressure across all three ages. The coefficient for change with age was inverse, but small and insignificant. In contrast, there was a significant effect of childhood social class on change in blood pressure with age, as well as on blood pressure at age 36 years. These effects of father's social class and birthweight were independent of each other, and adjusting for adult BMI at 36, 43 and 53 years strengthened the effect of birthweight on blood pressure but had no effect on the estimates for change. In contrast, after adjusting for adult BMI, the effect of childhood social class on the intercept was reduced and the effect on blood pressure change was substantially reduced and no longer significant. What is most interesting from the point of view of explaining inequalities in CHD risk is that the effect of father's social class on the adult blood pressure trajectory was mediated through its effects on the BMI trajectory.

In summary, there is little evidence to suggest that variation in size at birth explains childhood social class differentials in adult CHD risk. It is more likely that the BMI trajectory in later childhood or adult life mediates the effects of these social class differences. More research on lifetime BMI trajectories, and social class differences in these trajectories, in relation to CHD and its risk factors is necessary to develop these ideas further. Lifetime weight trajectories will vary by cohort, gender and place, related to the timing of the striking secular trends in childhood and adult weight gain observed in many European countries. This may result in more heterogeneity in social class differences in weight gain, particularly in childhood, than, say, in height growth. For example, childhood BMI change was apparently not strongly related to childhood social class in the Helsinki cohort. However, in other studies a strong effect of social class on childhood growth has been observed. For example, a study of three generations in Aberdeen (Morton 2002), showed that various measures of childhood growth, such as weight for height at age seven years, conditional on fetal growth, were strongly associated with parental social class. Some of this effect was explained by maternal characteristics such as maternal height, age, parity and hypertension, but social class effects remained after adjustment for these factors. This study also highlights the potential importance of inter-generational social class effects for adult CHD, operating through effects on maternal growth. Better socio-economic circumstances of the grandparents led to better childhood growth in the mother and eventually to higher birthweight in the subsequent generation, whereas poorer socio-economic circumstances in the grandparent's generation led to impaired childhood growth in the mothers, and lower birthweight in the subsequent generation (Morton 2002). These lower birthweights may, in turn, eventually affect this generation's risk of adult CHD (Barker 1998). Thus for a particular generation, their risk of CHD may be affected not only by their own socio-economic circumstances, but also by the circumstances of their grandparents and parents, but these effects may be mediated through different biological mechanisms. So while this does not alter the previous conclusion that size at birth is unlikely to account for childhood social differentials in CHD, it may account for any effects of grandparents' socio-economic circumstances on grandchildren's risk of CHD. This remains to be studied.

Contribution of neurodevelopmental factors to adult health

Neurodevelopmental factors offer another potential explanation for childhood socio-economic differences in adult health. Socially patterned exposures may impair childhood neurodevelopment. For example, there is growing evidence that early adverse social experiences can have lasting effects on stress reactivity in children (Boyce and Keating 2004). Other evidence points to associations between subtle deficits in thyroid hormone exposure prenatally or in the early postnatal period and subsequent neurodevelopmental deficits in childhood (Factor-Litvak and Susser 2004). The extent to which childhood neurodevelopmental deficits continue into adulthood with possible implications not just for neuropsychiatric outcomes but also for adult physical function and chronic disease is a growing area of life course research.

One way of investigating the link between neurodevelopment and adult physical function and chronic disease is to study childhood cognitive ability, and this information is available in a number of cohort studies. Early cognitive ability may provide a window on brain development, for example, acting as an indicator of the efficiency of information processing in the central nervous system. Numerous neuroendocrine, neuroanatomical, and neurochemical systems are involved in cognitive function and in the control of physical organ systems, some of which may have their origins in early life. There are striking social class differences in cognitive ability that strengthen through childhood and adolescence (Jefferis *et al.* 2003). Could early cognitive ability explain childhood socio-economic differences in adult health and disease?

There is growing evidence of an association between childhood cognitive ability and longevity (Hart *et al.* 2003, Kuh *et al.* 2004b, Osler *et al.* 2003, Whalley and Deary 2001). One study (Osler *et al.* 2003), using data from a Danish birth cohort born in 1953, showed that men with lower scores on IQ tests at age 12 had a higher risk of subsequent mortality. This study is interesting for our purposes because it also showed an effect of early childhood circumstances on later mortality and explicitly tested whether this could be accounted for by early cognitive ability or birthweight. Birthweight, while related to subsequent mortality, failed to be a mediating factor. Early ability was a far more important mediator. Childhood IQ mediated about a quarter of the effect of childhood socio-economic circumstances on all cause mortality. A study of the 1946 cohort also showed that higher male adult all-cause mortality was associated with lower childhood cognitive ability (Kuh *et al.* 2004b), and that childhood IQ mediated a similar proportion of the effect of childhood social class on mortality as it did in the Danish cohort study (unpublished data).

As yet, it is unclear whether the association between poor early cognitive ability and higher mortality risk is accounted for primarily by neurodevelopmental pathways, or social pathways given that early cognitive ability is also associated with safer adult environments and healthy adult behaviours (Whalley and Deary 2001). Studies from the Midspan cohort (Hart *et al.* 2003), and the 1946 cohort (Kuh *et al.* 2004b), suggest that a small effect of early ability remains after adjustment for adult socio-economic circumstances. Further studies of early ability and lifetime socio-economic circumstances in relation to specific diseases or functional outcomes are warranted.

Explanations for socio-economic differences in adult function

We know from cohort studies that midlife function is associated with current health and predicts subsequent disease, independence, disability and death. Many aspects of function are socially patterned but we must be cautious in delineating the temporal sequence of events and attributing cause and effect. Socio-economic conditions may initially affect function but poor function in turn may have an effect on subsequent socio-economic trajectories, which in turn have a further effect on functional trajectories. Despite these difficulties there are enormous benefits in studying functional trajectories. We may identify when early preventive action may be most effective. For example in the research on blood pressure and BMI weight trajectories discussed earlier we can observe periods either of accelerating risk, or of growing divergence between social groups.

There is a growing interest in simple tests of physical capability in elderly populations in order to study frailty and trajectories of functional decline. Some of these tests were used in the 1946 cohort when participants were aged 53. Strength was measured by hand grip using electronic dynamometers (Kuh *et al.* 2002a). Postural control was measured by a one-legged stand with eyes closed for up to 30 seconds, and less than 50 per cent of the cohort managed to do this for longer than five seconds (Kuh *et al.* 2005). Functional leg power was measured by 10 timed chair rises and the reciprocal of the time taken was used so that higher scores indicated better performance, just as they did in the other two tests. Using an aggregate standardized score of all three tests, and distinguishing those in the highest and lowest 10 per cent of this score, we showed that those brought up in the poorer circumstances had a higher risk of poor function at age 53 years (Guralnik *et al.*, in press). Conversely, those from more advantageous circumstances had a higher chance of good function. Adjusting for adult socio-economic conditions had hardly any effect on these relationships; adjusting for behavioural factors (smoking, exercise and alcohol consumption) and BMI explained some of the effect of childhood circumstances on poor function but not the effect on good function. To understand how the underlying pathways may account for these socio-economic differentials in physical capability it is best to study the individual components. To illustrate, we attempted to account for the child and the adult social class differentials in standing balance by a variety of factors, already identified as lifetime risk factors for poor standing balance. These include physical inactivity (Kuh *et al.*, 2005), lower lifetime cognitive ability and a lifetime weight trajectory characterized by poor weight gain in childhood and excess weight gain in adolescence and adult life (Kuh *et al.*, in press). About 10 per cent of the *childhood* social class differential in standing balance was explained by the lifetime weight trajectory (Figure 2.6a). Having taken this into account, childhood cognitive ability and educational attainment have strong effects, reducing the childhood social class differential by a further 40 per cent. After that, adjustment for adult physical activity, while strongly related to standing balance (Kuh *et al.*, 2005), resulted in a marginal reduction in the childhood social class differential. The lifetime weight trajectory explained none of the *adult* social class differential in standing balance, but cognitive ability and education remained strong explanations, and physical activity had a slightly more important effect in reducing the adult than the child social class differential (Figure 2.6b).

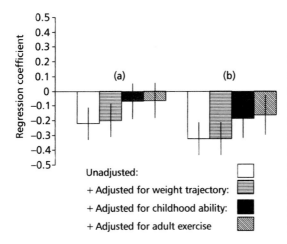

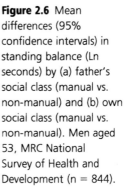

Figure 2.6 Mean differences (95% confidence intervals) in standing balance (Ln seconds) by (a) father's social class (manual vs. non-manual) and (b) own social class (manual vs. non-manual). Men aged 53, MRC National Survey of Health and Development (n = 844).

Unadjusted:

+ Adjusted for weight trajectory:

+ Adjusted for childhood ability:

+ Adjusted for adult exercise

Putting the risk factors into the regression model in a different order did not change the interpretation.

We also attempted to account for the childhood and adult social class differential in lung function observed in the 1946 cohort. Lung function, as measured by FEV1, is strongly related to respiratory disease and affected by biological and social factors operating at all stages of life. Like standing balance, it is strongly socially patterned. There was a reduction in both the childhood and adult social class differential in lung function of about 12 per cent after adjusting for developmental risk factors and early exposures. This group of risk factors includes lower childhood height and weight, infant chest illness, maternal smoking during childhood, and not being breast-fed (Wadsworth *et al.* 2004). Having taken account of these factors, adjusting for cognitive ability and education reduced both the child and adult social class differential considerably (by about two-fifths). Educational attainment and cognitive ability have independent effects on lung function despite being highly correlated (Richards *et al.* 2005). In addition, adult smoking and physical inactivity further reduced the coefficients, particularly for adult social class, and adult weight reduced the differentials a little more (see Figure 2.7).

In summary, it is not difficult at this level of explanation to account for the social class differentials in these aspects of adult function. We can 'explain' over 80 per cent of the childhood social differential in standing balance and

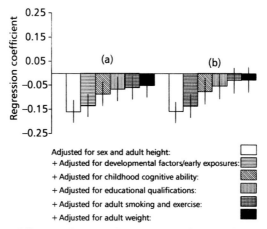

Figure 2.7 Mean differences (95% confidence intervals) in lung function (FEV1) by (a) father's social class (manual vs. non-manual) and (b) own social class (manual vs. non-manual). Men and women aged 53, MRC National Survey of Health and Development (n = 1967). Acknowledgements: MEJ Wadsworth, M Richards.

about 70 per cent of the adult differential if we know about physical and cognitive development, lifetime weight change and behavioural factors. To understand these associations at the next level of explanation, in terms of underlying biological mechanisms such as hormonal pathways, nutrition and lifetime disease exposure, will take further research. This presents a challenging and exciting research agenda.

Summary and future directions

In this chapter we have set out potential life course explanations for social inequalities in mortality, morbidity and function. We have outlined the conceptual basis for the influence of childhood circumstances on developmental trajectories, across physical and emotional, cognitive and social domains. Such conceptual models build on an extensive literature showing social patterning of key childhood developmental indicators. Their relevance to inequalities in adult health has been illustrated here for several adult outcomes that are likely to arise as a result of differing life course processes. Specifically, our examples suggest that the lifetime BMI trajectory is of particular relevance to the unequal development of cardiovascular outcomes and the lifetime weight trajectory is of relevance to inequalities in adult physical capability. These BMI and weight trajectories are affected by exposures acting from the early stages of life. Other examples illustrated in this chapter showed that neurodevelopmental pathways may be of relevance to inequality in adult physical capability, psychological distress and survival. Socio-emotional lifetime experiences were shown to be implicated in the development of inequalities in self reported health and psychological distress. We also acknowledge that health behaviours, particularly lifetime behavioural trajectories that are able to take timing and duration into account, will be of relevance for a broad range of health inequalities.

Research on life course and unequal health highlights the links between biological and social mechanisms. However, difficulties of capturing the sequential complexity in crude statistical models mean that caution is needed to avoid over-interpretation of findings. In this context, studies of functional trajectories (such as for blood pressure or lung function) rather than outcomes at just one point in time may be particularly informative.

Future studies aiming to understand the development of socio-economic health differentials are likely to build on several emerging themes in life course research. One central theme focuses on the timing and duration of influences on adult health and important transition points. Illustrating this approach is work that seeks to assess the relative importance of social class in childhood and adulthood, and also grandparental social class. The latter represents an extension of the time period being considered in which potentially relevant processes might be operating, and it signals inclusion of intergenerational effects in life course research.

A second major theme of future research will be the biological mechanisms that underlie the observed inequalities in health. A multiplicity of socially patterned exposures and intermediate mechanisms are likely to be involved. The biological processes considered in future work are likely to include interactions between genetic and environmental factors, as well as interactions between earlier and later life environmental influences. This research will also benefit from further study of functional trajectories, both as outcomes of these processes and then as exposures for chronic diseases.

A third theme emerging from recent research and likely to be developed in future work is the evaluation of heterogeneity of observations across disease, time and place. Studies comparing effects of social class in childhood across disease outcomes demonstrate the usefulness of this approach and there is also some recent comparative work on childhood class effects across populations born at different times and places (Galobardes *et al.* 2004, Power *et al.* 2005). This emerging theme on heterogeneity of effects is worthy of further investigation. Thus far however, comparison of life course influences across disease, time and place has relied primarily on reviews of published studies and there is scope for methodological developments in this area to formally evaluate differences observed. Study design and analysis will continue to be important themes in future work, influencing our ability to test conceptual life course models developed to investigate health inequalities.

Policy implications

Life course research to date suggests that, to a differing extent across health outcomes, inequality develops as a result of various socially patterned exposures and behaviours starting in early life through to later life stages. Thus, a life course approach cautions against 'single bullet' policies to improve inequalities. Rather, improving social inequalities in adult health requires a range of targeted intervention strategies for infants, children, adolescents and adults. In the early years of life these would include preschool and school intervention programmes designed to impact on developmental, social and behavioural as well as health trajectories (Keating and Hertzman 1999, Giles 2003). Testing life course models to identify the key pathways linking early life to adult health should highlight what interventions might be most effective for long-term health. The transition from adolescence to young adulthood offers another window of opportunity for interventions designed to break social and biological chains of risk and alter life course trajectories in ways that reduce subsequent health inequalities. Those socially or biologically disadvantaged from early life, for example, should receive extra help at this stage of life. Targeting interventions for young girls and women may improve not only their own health but also the health of future offspring. In adult life, we should continue to focus on known risk factors, such as smoking and obesity, because their contribution to health inequalities is firmly established (Aboderin *et al.* 2002). In addition to policies directed at different life stages, fiscal policies are needed that are designed to improve the distribution of living standards across the life course and across the population, given the growing evidence from life course studies of the long-term effects on health of growing up in poor socio-economic circumstances (Graham 2002, Giles 2003).

Finally, policies are needed that address macro-structural social, economic and cultural forces that encourage the uptake and maintenance of risk behaviours (Aboderin *et al.* 2002, Giles 2003). These include, for example, the reduction in advertising or positive cultural representations of smoking and unhealthy foods and the provision of low-cost sports and leisure facilities. In short, a life course approach to reduce inequalities in adult health calls for a combination of policies, those that focus on the pathways linking developmental and adult health and those that focus on the social, cultural and material conditions in which they are embedded (Graham and Power 2004).

Conclusions

Life course research on the development of unequal health has grown enormously in recent years, both in terms of conceptual evaluation and the extent of empirical investigation. In this chapter, our illustration of this body of research has relied heavily on observations from two well-characterized British birth cohort studies that have been studied intensively for the last half-century. Further comparison of research on life course influences on unequal health across these cohorts and in other populations will be crucial in revealing the extent to which findings from the two British cohorts, born in one country and only 12 years apart, are specific to their time and place. New studies are becoming established across Europe, Australia and North America and increased activity to construct longitudinal follow-up of old childhood studies and record linkage will promote further understanding of how inequalities in health develop over time and how these vary for different populations. The development of health inequalities over the life course will be elucidated by studying how social and physical contexts, biological vulnerability, and developmental processes operate together to modify functional trajectories and influence disease risk.

Acknowledgements

We thank Clive Osmond for providing unpublished analyses in Figure 2.5. Foremost, we are grateful to Hilary Graham for her input and support of the Life-course working group of the ESF program Social Variations in Health Expectancy in Europe.

References

Aboderin I, Kalache A, Ben-Shlomo Y *et al.* (2002). *Life course perspectives on coronary heart disease, stroke and diabetes: key issues and implications for policy and research.* World Health Organization, Geneva.

Barker DJP (1991). The foetal and infant origins of inequalities in health in Britain. *Journal of Public Health Medicine*, **13**, 64–8.

Barker DJP (1998). *Mothers, babies and health in later life*, 2nd edn, Churchill Livingstone, Edinburgh.

Ben-Shlomo Y and Kuh D (2002). A life course approach to chronic disease epidemiology: conceptual models, empirical challenges, and interdisciplinary perspectives. *International Journal of Epidemiology*, **31**, 285–93.

Boyce WT and Keating DP (2004). Should we intervene to improve childhood circumstances? In: D Kuh and Y Ben-Shlomo (eds) *A life course approach to chronic disease epidemiology*, 2nd edn, pp. 415–45. Oxford University Press, Oxford.

Brown GW and Harris TO (1978). *Social origin of depression.* Tavistock, London.

Davey Smith G, Gunnell D and Ben-Shlomo Y (2001). Life-course approaches to socio-economic differentials in cause-specific adult mortality. In: D Leon and G Walt (eds) *Poverty, inequality and health*, pp. 88–124. Oxford University Press, Oxford.

Davey Smith G, Hart C, Blane D and Hole D (1998). Adverse socio-economic conditions in childhood and cause specific adult mortality: prospective observational study. *British Medical Journal*, **316**, 1631–5.

Davey Smith G and Lynch J (2004). Life course approaches to socio-economic differentials in health. In: D Kuh and Y Ben-Shlomo (eds) *A life course approach to chronic disease epidemiology*, 2nd edn, pp. 77–115. Oxford University Press, Oxford.

Eriksson J, Forsen T, Tuomilehto J, Osmond C and Barker D (2004). Fetal and childhood growth and hypertension in adult life. *Hypertension*, **36**, 790–4.

Eriksson J, Forsen T, Tuomilehto J, Osmond C and Barker DJP (2001). Early growth and coronary heart disease in later life: longitudinal study. *British Medical Journal*, **322**, 949–53.

Factor-Litvak P and Susser E (2004). A life course approach to neuropsychiatric outcomes. In: D Kuh and Y Ben-Shlomo, eds. *A life course approach to chronic disease epidemiology*, 2nd edn, pp. 324–44. Oxford University Press, Oxford.

Ferri E, Bynner J and Wadsworth MEJ (2003). *Changing Britain: changing lives. Three generations at the turn of the century.* Bedford Way Press, London.

Fox J (1989). *Health inequalities in European countries.* Gower, Aldershot.

Galobardes B, Lynch JW and Davey Smith G (2004). Childhood socio-economic circumstances and cause-specific mortality in adulthood: systematic review and interpretation. *Epidemiologic Reviews*, **6**, 7–21.

Giles A (ed.) (2003). *A lifecourse approach to coronary heart disease prevention. Scientific and policy review.* National Heart Forum, The Stationery Office.

Gliksman MD, Kawachi I, Hunter D *et al.* (1995). Childhood socio-economic status and risk of cardiovascular disease in middle aged US women: a prospective study. *Journal of Epidemiology and Community Health*, **49**, 10–15.

Graham H (2002). Building an inter-disciplinary science of health inequalities: the example of lifecourse research. *Social Science and Medicine*, **55**, 2005–16.

Graham H and Power C (2004). *Childhood disadvantage and adult health: a lifecourse framework.* Health Development Agency, London.

Guralnik J, Butterworth S, Wadsworth MEJ, Kuh D. Childhood socioeconomic status predicts physical functioning a half century later. *J Gerontology (Medical Sciences).*

Hardy R, Kuh D, Langenberg C and Wadsworth MEJ (2003). Birthweight, childhood social class, and change in adult blood pressure in the 1946 British birth cohort. *Lancet*, **362**, 1178–83.

Hardy R, Wadsworth MEJ and Kuh D (2000). The influence of childhood weight and socio-economic status on change in adult body mass index in a British national birth cohort. *International Journal of Obesity*, **24**, 1–10.

Hart CL, Taylor MD, Davey Smith GDS *et al.* (2003). Childhood IQ, social class, deprivation, and their relationships with mortality and morbidity risk in later life: prospective observational study linking the Scottish Mental Survey 1932 and the Midspan Studies. *Psychosomatic Medicine*, **65**, 877–83.

Idler EL and Benyamini Y (1997). Self-rated health and mortality: a review of twenty-seven community studies. *Journal of Health and Social Behaviour*, **38**, 21–37.

Jefferis BJ, Graham H, Manor O and Power C (2003). Level of cigarette smoking and socio-economic circumstances in adolescence: how do they affect adult smoking? *Addiction*, **98**, 1765–72.

Keating D and Hertzman C (1999). *Developmental health and the wealth of nations: social, biological and educational dynamics.* The Guilford Press, New York.

Kuh D, Bassey EJ, Butterworth S, Hardy R and Wadsworth MEJ (2005). Grip strength, postural control and functional leg power in a representative cohort of middle-aged British men and women: associations with current and previous physical activity and health status, and socio-economic conditions. *Journal of Gerontology (Medical Sciences)*, **60A**, 224–31.

Kuh D, Bassey EJ, Hardy R, Aihie Sayer A, Wadsworth M and Cooper C (2002a) Birthweight, childhood size and muscle strength in adult life: evidence from a birth cohort study. *American Journal of Epidemiology*, **156**, 627–33.

Kuh D and Ben-Shlomo Y (2004). *A life course approach to chronic disease epidemiology: tracing the origins of ill-health from early to adult life*, 2nd edn. Oxford University Press, Oxford.

Kuh D, Ben-Shlomo Y, Lynch J, Hallqvist J and Power C (2003). A glossary for life course epidemiology. *Journal of Epidemiology and Community Health*, **57**, 778–83.

Kuh D and Hardy R (2002). *A life course approach to women's health.* Oxford University Press, Oxford.

Kuh D, Hardy R, Langenberg C, Richards M and Wadsworth MEJ (2002b). Mortality in adults aged 26–54 years related to socio-economic conditions in childhood and adulthood: a post war birth cohort study. *British Medical Journal*, **325**, 1076–80.

Kuh D, Power C, Blane D and Bartley M (2004a). Socio-economic pathways between childhood and adult health. In: D Kuh and Y Ben-Shlomo (eds) *A life course approach to chronic disease epidemiology*, 2nd edn, pp. 371–98. Oxford University Press, Oxford.

Kuh D, Richards M, Hardy R, Butterworth S and Wadsworth MEJ (2004b). Childhood cognitive ability and deaths up until middle age: a post war birth cohort study. *International Journal of Epidemiology*, **33**, 408–13.

Kuh D, Hardy R, Butterworth S, Okell L, Richards M, Wadsworth MEJ, Cooper C, Aihie Sayer A. Developmental origins of midlife performance: evidence from a British birth cohort (*Am J Epidemid*).

Kunst A, Groenhof F, Mackenbach J and EU Working Group on socio-economic Inequalities in Health (1998). Occupational class and cause specific mortality in middle aged men in 11 European countries: comparison of population-based studies. *British Medical Journal*, **316**, 1636–42.

Lawlor DA, Ben-Shlomo Y and Leon DA (2004). Pre-adult influences on cardiovascular disease. In: D Kuh and Y Ben-Shlomo (eds) *A life course approach to chronic disease epidemiology*, 2nd end, pp. 41–76. Oxford University Press, Oxford.

Lawlor DA, Ebrahim S, Davey Smith G (2002). A life course approach to coronary heart disease and stroke. In: D Kuh and R Hardy (eds) *A life course approach to women's health*. Oxford University Press, Oxford.

Li L, Manor O and Power C (2004) Early environment and child-to-adult growth trajectories in the 1958 British birth cohort. *American Journal of Clinical Nutrition*, **80**, 185–92.

Mackenbach JP, Kunst AE, Cavelaars AE, Groenhof F, Guerts JJ and the EU Working Group on socio-economic Inequalities in Health (1997). Socio-economic inequalities in morbidity and mortality in middle-aged men in western Europe. *Lancet*, **349**, 1655–9.

Marmot MG, Shipley MJ and Rose G (1984). Inequalities in death – specific explanations of a general pattern? *Lancet*, 5 May 1003–6.

Maughan B and McCarthy G (1997). Childhood adversities and psychosocial disorders. In M Marmot and M Wadsworth (eds) *Fetal and early child environment: long-term health implications*, pp. 156–69. British Medical Bulletin.

Morton S (2002). Life course determinants of offspring size at birth: an intergenerational study of Aberdeen women. London, Unpublished PhD thesis.

Osler M, Andersen AM, Due P, Lund R, Damsgaard MT and Holstein BE (2003). Socio-economic position in early life, birth weight, childhood cognitive function, and adult mortality. A longitudinal study of Danish men born in 1953. *Journal of Epidemiology and Community Health*, **57**, 681–6.

Power C and Matthews S (1997). Origins of health inequalities in a national population sample. *Lancet*, **350**, 1584–9.

Power C, Graham H, Due P *et al.* (2005). The contribution of childhood and adult socio-economic position to adult obesity and smoking behaviour: an international comparison. *International Journal of Epidemiology*, **34**, 335–44.

Power C, Manor O and Matthews S (2003). Child to adult socio-economic conditions and obesity in a national cohort. *International Journal of Obesity*, **27**, 1081–6.

Power C, Manor O and Matthews S (1999). The duration and timing of exposure: effects of socio-economic environment on adult health. *American Journal of Public Health*, **89**, 1059–65.

Power C, Matthews S and Manor O (1998). Inequalities in self-rated health: explanations from different stages of life. *Lancet*, **351**, 1009–14.

Power C, Stansfeld SA, Matthews S, Manor O and Hope S (2002). Childhood and adulthood risk factors for socio-economic differentials in psychological distress: evidence from the 1958 British birth cohort. *Social Science and Medicine*, **55**, 1989–2004.

Richards M, Strachan D, Hardy R, Kuh D and Wadsworth MEJ (2005). Lung function and cognitive ability in a longitudinal birth cohort study. *Psychosomatic Medicine*, **67**, 602–8.

Robins LN (1978). Sturdy childhood predictors of adult antisocial behaviour: replications from longitudinal studies. *Psychological Medicine*, **8**, 611–22.

Strachan D and Sheikh A (2004). A life course approach to respiratory and allergic diseases. In: D Kuh and Y Ben-Shlomo (eds) *A life course approach to chronic disease epidemiology*, 2nd edn, pp. 240–59. Oxford University Press, Oxford.

Van de Mheen H, Stronks S and Mackenback JP (1998). A lifecourse perspective on socio-economic inequalities in health: the influence of childhood socio-economic conditions and selection processes. *Sociology of Health and Illness*, **20**, 754–77.

Wadsworth M, Vinall LE, Jones AL *et al.* (2004). Alpha-1-antitrypsin as a risk for infant and adult respiratory outcomes in a national birth cohort. *American Journal of Respiratory cell and Molecular Biology*, **31**, 559–64.

Whalley LJ and Deary IJ (2001). Longitudinal cohort study of childhood IQ and survival up to age 76. *British Medical Journal*, **322**, 1–5.

Chapter 3

The shape of things to come

How social policy impacts social integration and family structure to produce population health

Lisa F. Berkman and Maria Melchior

Introduction

Population health rests largely on shaping the distribution of risk in a population so that fewer people are exposed to risky situations. To a lesser extent, we are interested in reducing the relative risks related to exposures though we have a clear and primary role in identifying the magnitude of such risks. Over the last 30 to 40 years a massive amount of evidence has accumulated about what we now call 'social determinants of health' (Rose 1992, Berkman and Kawachi 2000). This volume is dedicated to describing this evidence and the newest directions in which scientists are moving.

Our aim is somewhat different. We hope to start to move the field of population health from drawing almost exclusively on observational studies to describe the adverse impacts of social conditions on health to (1) understand how observational studies can lead to evidence-based policy and (2) to evaluate the effects of specific policies on population health using experimental or quasi-experimental designs (Cook and Campbell 1979, Cook 2002). In this chapter, we draw on our work on social integration and social relations to illustrate new approaches. We also find it useful to use cross-country comparisons in this work. Most of the work we build on in the chapter is based on comparisons between the US and France. We are particularly concerned with the interface between economic inequality and social integration across the countries and the ways in which public and private sector social and economic policies serve to shape or promote cultural values regarding family and work in the two countries. We are aware that in many ways France shares political positions and cultural values with other western European countries and may not be 'unique' in its social policy approaches. Looking across industrialized countries, especially those in the

OECD, it is more likely that the US is an outlier in many regards than that France is in a truly unique position. However, in this chapter we use France and the US as case studies to illustrate our points. We think it is valuable to build on a cross-country comparison between the US and France with regard to social relationships, social policy and health. Our hope is that this chapter will incite more work in this area. The work serves as the initial step on a pathway.

In the following pages we will (1) briefly review the evidence linking social networks to health outcomes, primarily mortality, across countries with special attention to data from the US and France; (2) discuss the interface between economic inequality and social integration; and (3) explore whether patterns of social integration can explain population health at the country level. Finally, we discuss social and economic policies that may promote health and positive social relationships especially with regard toward work and family issues.

The link between social networks and health

The way social networks are structured and the functions and resources that flow from those networks have profound effects on health and behaviour (Berkman and Glass 2000). Furthermore, relationships have a valence – they can be positive, intimate, nurturing, supportive, etc. or negative – conflicted, demeaning, hostile (Rook 1992, Kiecolt-Glaser et al. 1997). Depending upon the structure, function and valence of these relations, networks can be health-promoting or damaging. Networks influence health outcomes based on these structures and functions which in turn provide opportunities for support, influence, social engagement, access to resources and material goods and through person-to-person contact transmit infectious diseases.

For these reasons, the study of social networks and health has become much more nuanced over the last years, with a deeper probing of structural configurations at the macro-level (Bearman et al. 2004) and an understanding of the complex dynamics between dyadic pairs (partners, parents-children, employers-employees). For lengthier reviews of this topic, the reader is referred to Berkman et al. (2000), Cohen (2004), Kiecolt-Glaser et al. (1997) and Marsden and Friedkin (1994). In this chapter we will discuss dimensions of networks related to overall levels of social integration. We focus on these dimensions because we suspect they are most likely to be influenced by macro-social and structural conditions, social and economic policies, and cultural values at country levels.

A number of studies in the US, UK, Scandinavia and Japan have shown that indices of social integration or participation are associated with all-cause mortality, and generally most strongly with mortality from cardiovascular disease (Berkman and Syme 1979, House *et al.* 1982, Blazer 1982, Orth-Gomer and Johnson 1987, Sugisawa *et al.* 1994). These studies generally assess integration by ties in several domains: marriage or stable partnerships, ties with close friends and relatives, participation in voluntary and/or civic associations and membership in a religious organization. With few exceptions, the analyses have not been conducted in countries in western and southern Europe where it is often thought that social cohesion is high and both familial and community ties are valued. In fact, work in this area started in large part to illustrate how the social fragmentation and exclusion evident in the US might have dramatic effects on health and well-being.

We conducted an analysis in France among a large cohort of French employees of Electricity of France – Gas of France (EDF-GDF) known as the GAZEL cohort to test whether social isolation would predict increased mortality risk in a French cohort of middle-aged men and women who were stably employed in a large public company (Berkman *et al.* 2004). The study in this French cohort had both advantages and disadvantages. The advantages were that it would test the hypothesis in a large middle-aged sample of men and women across a diverse range of grades of employment from manual workers to managers. Second, most studies of social networks and health have been studied in populations where cardiovascular disease is the major cause of death. Cancer is a leading cause of death among middle-aged and older people in France. This study represented an opportunity to test the association between social isolation and death from cancer and other causes besides cardiovascular disease. Finally, France is a country where contacts with family members are high, and nationally representative data indicate that family contacts (Pan Ke Shon 1999) are more common in France than in the US. Some of the disadvantages of the study are related to the fact that any occupational cohort is a selected and truncated population, likely to exclude the most isolated members of the population, those who are unable to work, and those with few skills or training to enter into the occupation. Furthermore, in this study, physical exams were not conducted so we have limited information on biological pathways or mediating mechanisms linking our exposures to mortality.

In 1989, EDF-GDF and the French National Institute of Health and Medical Research launched the longitudinal cohort of EDF-GDF employees. EDF-GDF employs approximately 150,000 people across a diversified set of trades and in a very wide range of employment grades. The profile of the cohort is close to the general population of France in many respects (Chevalier *et al.* 1987) although everyone is employed. Ages of employees are truncated at high and low ages (participants were aged 35 to 50 at study baseline). Items on social integration were added on the 1991 survey and analyses presented here are based on 16,699 participants who responded in that year (83.6 per cent of the original cohort). Mortality data are available from the baseline interview through 1999. There were 281 deaths among men and 46 among women occurring during this period. Because we were concerned that illness at baseline might influence social participation, we excluded deaths occurring in the first two years of follow-up, reducing our events to 228 and 29 among men and women respectively.

A social integration index was adapted from the Alameda County Study (Berkman and Syme 1979) to be appropriate for the current French study. The index assesses contact or ties in three domains which are each scored 0–2: (1) marital status or cohabitation, (2) contacts with close friends and family, (3) affiliation with voluntary associations. Level 1 of the index includes persons who scored 0 or 1 and levels II, III, IV include those who scored 2–3, 4–5, and 6 respectively. The reader is referred to the original publication for further details (Berkman et al. 2004).

The distribution of specific domains of the index as well as the overall score are shown on Table 3.1 along with other relevant socio-demographic data. The distribution of scores is different for men and women with women less likely to be married or cohabiting, having slightly fewer ties with friends and relatives and less likely to belong to voluntary organizations. This is subsequently reflected in the range of scores in the summary index. However, by far the most notable finding is that 1.4 per cent of men and 6.8 per cent of women fall into the most isolated category. We will return to a further discussion of this finding.

With regard to the risk associated with levels of social integration, Figure 3.1 shows the multivariate adjusted relative risks for men and women in relation to all-cause mortality. Men with the fewest ties have a Risk Ratio (RR) of 2.70, Confidence Interval (CI) 1.17 – 6.23 of dying compared to those with the most ties. There is a steady gradient in risk with decreasing connections. Among women the relative risk is 3.64 (CI .72-18.58), which is not significant in all likelihood due to the small number of deaths among women in the cohort. Tests for trends across the categories are significant for both men (p = 0.0006) and women (p = 0.012).

We were then interested in testing whether social connectedness was associated with similar or different causes of death in France as compared with the US, UK and much of Scandinavia. Table 3.2 shows the age-adjusted and multivariate risks for mortality from cancer, cardiovascular disease and accidents and suicide for men in the GAZEL cohort. The small number of

Table 3.1 Demographic, social and health-related characteristics of GAZEL participants in 1991

	Men (n = 12,347)	Women (n = 4,352)
Year of birth		
1949–1953	–	39.1 (1701)
1944–1949	57.8 (7133)	36.1 (1572)
1939–1944	42.2 (5214)	24.8 (1079)
Occupational grade		
Unskilled	11.8 (1447)	23.1 (1003)
Skilled	54.6 (6723)	66.7 (2892)
Manager	33.6 (4141)	10.2 (441)
Marital status		
Married/cohabitating	92.7 (11426)	77.2 (3348)
Single/never married	2.3 (280)	7.2 (313)
Widowed/divorced	5.0 (619)	15.6 (677)
Numbers of contacts		
0–2	6.1 (749)	8.7 (378)
3–11	41.2 (5088)	52.7 (2293)
> 11	52.7 (6510)	38.6 (1681)
Group membership		
0	24.0 (2962)	38.9 (1692)
1	37.8 (4670)	35.1 (1526)
≥ 2	38.2 (4715)	26.1 (1134)
Social integration		
IV (high)	21.3 (2632)	9.1 (397)
III	58.4 (7208)	48.6 (2117)
II	18.9 (2336)	35.5 (1543)
I (low)	1.4 (171)	6.8 (295)
Mortality		
% died	2.3 (281)	1.1 (46)

deaths in women prohibited these refined analyses by cause of death for women. For cancer mortality, the relative risks in multivariate models ranged from 3.60 for the least integrated men to 2.17 and 1.47 for men in increasingly integrated categories (test for trend = 0.0089). Cardiovascular risks associated were not significant and ranged from 1.29 for those in the most isolated

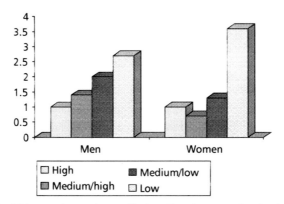

Figure 3.1 Social integration and mortality in a French occupational cohort: EDF-GDF employees. Adjusted for age, occupational grade, cigarette smoking, alcohol consumption, BMI, depressive symptoms, self-rated health, and geographical region.

Table 3.2 Age-adjusted and multivariate relative risks of mortality from cancer, cardiovascular disease, and accidents and suicide among men in the GAZEL cohort, by level of social integration, France, 1993–1999.

Cause of death and social integration index	Age-adjusted model*		Fully adjusted model†	
	RR‡	95% CI‡	RR	95% CI
Cancer	(n = 96)		(n = 90)	
IV (high)	1		1	
III	1.6	0.9, 3.1	1.5	0.8, 2.8
II	2.5	1.3, 5.0	2.2	1.1, 4.3
I (low)	5.3	1.7, 6.4	3.6	1.0,13.0
p for trend	0.0008		0.0089	
Cardiovascular disease	(n = 50)		(n = 47)	
IV (high)	1		1	
III	1.0	0.5, 2.1	1.0	0.5, 2.3
II	1.3	0.5, 3.0	1.1	0.5, 2.8
I (low)	1.6	0.2, 12.5	1.3	0.2,10.4
p for trend	0.5		0.7	
Accidents and suicide	(n = 41)		(n = 40)	
IV (high)	1		1	
III	1.1	0.4, 2.6	0.9	0.3, 2.4
II	3.1	1.2, 7.8	2.7	1.1, 7.0
I (low)	5.4	1.1, 26.7	3.5	0.7,18.4
p for trend	0.0012		0.0053	

* Adjusted for age only.

† Adjusted for age, occupational grade, cigarette smoking, alcohol consumption, body mass index, depressive symptoms, self-rated health, and geographic region of France.

‡ RR, relative risk; CI, confidence interval.

categories to 1.13 and 1.07 for those more integrated men. The risks of dying of accidents or suicides show a significant test for trend ($p = 0.0053$) with risks ranging from 3.54 to 2.74 for those least integrated.

The finding that social integration is related to cancer mortality, the leading cause of death in middle-aged French men and women, is noteworthy and deserves further thought. In our study, social isolation was related to cancer mortality even when we controlled for tobacco and alcohol use and body mass index which in themselves are powerful predictors of cancer outcomes in the cohort (Melchior *et al.* 2005, Zins *et al.* 2003). Thus it seems likely that other pathways involving physiologic factors related to stressful exposures, or other environmental or behavioural factors unmeasured in this study may mediate this relationship. Our findings suggest that risk associated with social isolation may, to some extent, reflect patterns of disease distribution in the population and be culture and time-specific. Similar disease-specific patterns have been observed regarding socio-economic gradients in morbidity and mortality (Fuhrer *et al.* 2002, Leclerc *et al.* 1990). For instance, at times or in places where infectious diseases are rampant, economic gradients in these causes of morbidity and mortality are observed. It seems likely that these general patterns of association are the result of disease-specific pathways that wax and wane over time and across places (e.g. water purification, vaccines, and other medical interventions) as well as biological pathways likely to mediate multiple diseases (neuroendocrine responses, immune and metabolic responses) (Link and Phelan 1995). Efforts to identify the biologic, behavioural and psychological pathways that may link social experiences to cancer mortality in France and cardiovascular mortality in the US will help us understand variations in population health across countries. Disease distributions vary across time and place for a number of reasons, but social conditions create risky environments which in turn create vulnerable subgroups of the population who may be both more susceptible to other specific exposures and/or be more heavily exposed to a range of environmental risks. The two are not at all mutually exclusive and may in fact be reinforcing. A critical issue remains understanding the pathways by which social conditions influence health. Understanding cross-country variations is essential to this endeavour.

How is economic inequality linked to social isolation?

Structural and economic conditions provide both opportunities and barriers to maintaining social ties. Social networks also provide opportunities and barriers to social and economic advancement. For instance, early work on networks illustrated how networks predicted how people found jobs. These bidirectional influences make it difficult to sort out under what conditions causal patterns operate. Further complicating our understanding of these issues is that most of the empirical work in this area draws heavily on cross-sectional analyses, making it difficult to infer directionality. We might easily conceive however that economic conditions of disadvantage, poverty, and insecurity destroy relationships. In fact, inequality in many European countries defined in relative terms now as Wilkinson (2005) notes may have a significant impact in terms of 'social exclusion' of the poor. Economic circum-stances produce patterns of social exclusion by limiting an individual's ability to participate in work, family and community life. Conversely, there has been a body of work showing the structure of social networks is linked to finding jobs and gaining access to a number of resources (Granovetter 1973), thereby impacting economic opportunities.

Our aim in this chapter is not to parse the directionality of these two complex experiences but to explore whether the association between them varies across countries. Our hypothesis is that there is considerable variabil-ity in the magnitude of this association – the degree to which they are 'coupled'. For instance, Wilkinson in his work on the impact of inequality pro-poses that in egalitarian societies, to some extent regardless of the absolute levels of deprivation, social relations take a different form. They are less hos-tile, discriminatory and authoritarian and friendlier with higher levels of cooperation and sharing. Here we are concerned with a rather simpler ques-tion: Is the strength of the association between socio-economic position and social networks and family structure similar across settings, in this case across France and the US?

If we compare social network scores by socio-economic position in the Alameda County Study in the US and by occupational grade in the GAZEL study, we see different patterns. Among men in the US, about 25 per cent of upper SES men score in isolated categories whereas over 50 per cent of men and 70 per cent of women in the least advantaged positions are socially isolated (Berkman and Breslow 1983). In the US socio-economic position is associated with marital status, single parenthood, and participation in a range of voluntary and civic associations. Contact with close friends and relatives show weaker patterns of association, as does religious participation. Using a very similar index in the GAZEL cohort, we find much weaker associations between occupational grade and levels of social integration. There are virtually no differences between skilled workers and managers (among men in both groups, 1 per cent are socially isolated, about 6 per cent among women). Among unskilled workers, social isolation is more prevalent (2 per cent for men, 9 per cent for women). Of course, the major problem with this comparison is that the two cohorts are not completely similar. The Alameda County study was completed decades earlier and is a population-based study including men and women both in and out of the labour force. The scales are not identical, the GAZEL study is restricted to employees of EDF-GDF. Still, comparisons between GAZEL and the Whitehall Study of British Civil Servants (Fuhrer *et al.* 2002) suggest that occupation is differentially associated with a range of behavioural risk factors in the two cohorts with occupational grade being more strongly associated with risk in the UK than in France. Data from the French National Statistics Institute (INSEE) on representative samples of the French population show a more complex picture of socio-economic position and social ties. On the one hand those in the highest occupational grades (executives and professionals) have slightly smaller family networks (20 members on average) than skilled and unskilled workers (25 and 26), farmers (24), other-employed men and women (22). However, managers and professionals are more likely than unskilled workers to receive material or emotional support from members of their networks (Herpin and Dechaux 2004). Also, members of higher status groups are more likely than unskilled workers to belong to voluntary groups (61 compared to 29 per cent) (INSEE 2003). Overall, some other data suggest that extreme social isolation (measured as fewer than three personal contacts in the preceding week) is more frequent among the least educated (11.2 per cent), compared to the overall rate (16.5 per cent) (Pan Ke Shon 2003). Other indicators of social integration, such as voting patterns, also vary by socio-economic position (in 2004 French regional elections, the turnout was 71 per cent among university graduates, 67 per cent among high school graduates, 61 per cent among those with primary education, and 57 per cent among those without formal education) (INSEE 2004), but overall, voting participation is higher than in the United States (64 per cent in France compared to 60.7 per cent in the 2004 US Presidential election and 54.3 per cent in the 2000 Presidential elections) (Committee 2005). Labour markets, economic pressures and organizational relations certainly influence the structure of networks. Our data suggest that the association between socio-economic position and social networks, however, may not be identical across countries, because the nature of social relationships and the prevalence of social isolation do vary cross-culturally. The data however are not strictly comparable and further work in this area would be important. If economic conditions and networks are not inextricably coupled together in all societies, it would help us better understand the determinants of population health. Just as economic inequality among states in the US may be more strongly associated with adverse outcomes than inequality in other countries (Ross *et al.* 2005), so societies may differ in the value they place on the social bonds among family and community.

Do patterns of social integration and social exclusion shape population health?

Our proposition is that population health is shaped by a number of social and environmental conditions. Economic, environmental, social and health systems figure prominently in this model. Population health itself is based on both mean or average levels of health as well as the distribution of health. To date, researchers have focused predominantly on the role of economic circumstances and inequality in shaping patterns of population health. We agree that this focus on economic conditions is of the utmost importance and deserves critical attention. However, we also hypothesize that patterns of social integration, exclusion and network structure impact population health in important ways. Patterns of family formation shape child health and development and care-giving capacities for both children and adult dependents. On one hand they provide opportunities for intimacy, attachment and a sense of trust and belonging. On the other hand, networks can promote discrimination, conflict, hostility and exclusion. Social networks operate by regulating an individual's access to life-opportunities both emotional and material, by facilitating diffusion of influence and information and by providing opportunities for mobility (Granovetter 1973). Networks also shape the spread of disease transmission by patterns of social mixing.

Because there is so little evidence on networks across countries that is truly comparable, we pose the investigation of this issue as an important one for the future. Here we provide some evidence on patterns of contact among French families, voluntary associations, and civic participation as they relate to both social integration and exclusion vis-à-vis current patterns of immigration. We present this as a small case study of France with the hope it will stimulate stronger cross-national work.

Life expectancy (LE) in France is relatively high, especially for women. Compared with the US, French men and women live 1.3 and 3.4 years longer respectively. Among OECD countries, life expectancy for French women ranks near the very top with only Japan consistently having higher LE. For men France ranks 16 among 30 countries (OECD 2001). The US ranks 21 among 30 countries for overall LE. Rates of cardiovascular disease are especially low in France, leading to what is often called the French Paradox. Table 3.3 shows the number of contacts that adults in France have with their family members. French adults average 86 visits and 85 phone calls per year to their mothers. Assuming these are not on the same day, French adults have contact with their parents every other day of the year (171/356 days). French grandparents visit with their grandchildren on average 48 times a year (almost weekly). While there are not strictly comparable data in the US, visits and calls are much less

Table 3.3 Contacts among French family members. Number of meetings and telephone calls per year (PVC, 1997, 8000 households).

	Visits	**Calls**
Mother	86	85
Father	69	58
Child	85	66
Grandchild	48	–
Maternal grandparents	39	–
Paternal grandparents	25	–
Niece/nephew	37	–
Brother/sister	35	28

frequent. A European comparison conducted in 1994 showed that social isolation (measured by contacts with family and friends, membership in clubs and associations and social activity in the neighbourhood) is less frequent in France and other southern European countries than northern Europe (Paugam 1999). We are currently analyzing data from the European Social Survey to obtain some estimates across European countries.

At the same time, France is similar to the US in past patterns of immigration. France experienced a big wave of immigration around 1930 and then again in the 1970s – since the 1930s immigrants constitute about 7 per cent of France's population (Dagnet and Thave 1996). These immigrants came from southern and eastern Europe as well as former French colonies in northern Africa. French social policy through much of the later part of the twentieth century was oriented to helping immigrants adapt to French language and culture at the same time as they maintained cultural orientation to their country of immigration. After the Second World War, France's secular orientation hoped to protect citizens from discrimination based on religion or ethnicity.

France, like many European countries as well as the US and UK, now faces a new challenge from recent waves of immigration. Experience of social exclusion and discrimination appear to be growing and this may manifest itself in terms of population health (Bouvier-Colle *et al.* 1985). Using France as a case study may show us that if our proposition is correct, the way in which France responds to these recent waves of immigration will have substantial consequences in terms of population health.

The migrant population in France was traditionally based on needs for manual labour and was largely composed of men (Danzon *et al.* 1998). Since the mid 1970s, however, immigration patterns have been based more on the unification of families and exile from countries of origin outside of Europe. It has also become a population composed of almost equal numbers of men and women. By 1990 almost 45 per cent of immigrants were women. In the last several decades, immigrants to France came from sub-Saharan Africa and Southeast Asia (Danzon *et al.* 1998). Unlike many earlier waves of immigrants with European Judeo-Christian backgrounds, recent immigrants often from Muslim backgrounds and cultures with much less in common with traditional French culture find social integration in France much more challenging. Juggling multiple cultures in this instance when immigrants confront discrimination, find housing and education systems inappropriate to the values from their country of origin and/or religion, creates a situation of social exclusion. In 1999, immigrants represented 8.1 per cent of the French workforce, a majority working in unskilled jobs (69.2 per cent compared to of the workforce overall 55.6 per cent) (Thave 2000). Immigrants are also more likely to be unemployed (in 2004, 17.4 per cent compared to 9.2 per cent among no immigrants). This tension is particularly apparent in young adolescents and second-generation immigrants as they risk being rejected or excluded from both French communities and the immigrant networks based on country of origin (De Carmoy 1993).

Immigration policies regarding 'adaptation' in the French school system or work training programs that developed in France after the Second World War, may or may not turn out to be adaptive with new waves of immigrants. In any case, our aim here is not to provide clear answers to these challenges but to frame social integration and social exclusion as two sides of the same coin and propose that they have major consequences for the shaping of population health. We propose that both public and private sector policies as well as deeply entrenched cultural values about social participation will serve to shape patterns of health not only for the immigrants but because the 'contextual' spill-over into many social forums will influence the health of non-immigrants as well.

Do social and economic policies shape the structure of social networks?

Social and economic policies concerning immigration, housing, labour and education are not often developed with the aim of creating strong community and family bonds and promoting high levels of social integration and cohesion. There are however a number of policies in place, especially in western Europe, designed to ensure child well-being, especially in the face of poverty. Many of those programmes have shielded children successfully from the most severe forms of deprivation and abuse. As Barbara Bergman has noted, the US and France stand in stark contrast to one another on this issue and while French policies are similar to others in western Europe, they serve as a solid example of a particularly generous set of programmes to strengthen the security, health and development of French children (Bergmann 1996). Thus, a brief examination of French social policies suggests that France not only supports children through family-based and work-based policies, but in fact in many ways can be viewed as a country that is 'relationship-friendly'.

We suggest that these family and relationship-friendly policies promote the health of children, but also contribute to the health of French women whose life expectancy is among the highest in the world. In fact, LE for French women ranks consistently above most countries in the world except for Japan. LE for men, on the other hand, ranks in about the middle of OECD. Our preliminary findings suggest that economic and work-based policies put in place in France to maintain family and child health may have benefits for women, especially those in the workforce. We hope to explore this working hypothesis further in analyses that employ stronger analytic approaches and experimental and quasi-experimental designs. To date, few studies have used experimental or quasi-experimental designs to evaluate the health effects of social policies although there is a clear indication that such evidence-based policy may be informative (Cook 2002, Cook and Campbell 1979, Heymann 2000).

Some of France's impetus to develop programmes to support families with children grows from its pronatalist culture (Pedersen 1993). In response to low birth rates, France developed early policies to encourage couples to have large families – even today, for instance, pronatalist policies send disproportionately more benefits to families with three or more children (Bergmann 1996).

In many ways we can consider the social policies that France has developed as not only 'pro-family' but in a deeper sense, pro-relationships. The policies, some of which we outline below, serve families with young children as well as provide opportunities to care for dependents at the end of life. Here we list a series of French benefit programmes which we hypothesize impact the health of children and women. Future research in this area must strive to evaluate these programmes effectively. Here we simply identify some of the programmes we suspect are most important.

1 Family allowances: The social security system administers allowances to families with more than one child. When a woman is pregnant, she also receives a new baby allowance. Many but not all benefits are not income-tested. For low-income families with one child, benefits are available from other programmes. Other programmes provide assistance to single parents.

2 Day care and nursery school: Child-care expenses include both out-of-pocket expenses as well as publicly available crèches near many worksites and schools. Virtually all French children by the time they are three attend the *école maternelle*, a nursery school that enrols children during the entire day.

3 Family leave: Each parent has a right to parental leave for children $\leq$ three for one year, total or partial. Employee contract is maintained but not salary. Maternal leave is 16 weeks for 1–2 children and 26 weeks for $\geq$ three children with full salary paid by social security. There is an end of life leave to attend to a dependent for up to three months. Family event leave permits employees paid leave for other people's weddings, births, and funerals.

4 Work and vacation/sickness absence: French employees have five weeks paid vacation per year. In 2000, the legal duration of work was reduced to 35 hours per week. Fifty percent of wages are paid for 4–11 days of sickness. Pay is related to length of absence over 12 days.

Workplace practices and policies in the US are much more limited generally in both their actual benefits and practices concerning work/family balance. There is increasing evidence that not only care-giving related to children but also care-giving related to others can have important health effects (Schulz and Beach 1999). In a study we recently completed, middle-aged women (46–71) who cared for a disabled or ill spouse for $\geq$ nine hours a week had an almost twofold risk of coronary heart disease (CHD) (Lee *et al.* 2003). Tensions between work and home life exist for virtually all men and women in the workforce but they are likely to be especially acute for those with limited economic resources or insecure jobs. Since women assume many informal care-giving responsibilities, disadvantaged women may experience greatly increased risks. For example, Frankenhauser showed that employed women exhibited continual neuroendocrine activation at home in the evening, as opposed to men's drop (Frankenhaeuser *et al.* 1989, Frankenhaeuser 1989), potentially reflective of women's 'second shift'. Another investigation indicated that employed women with at least one child at home excreted significantly more urinary cortisol and reported more home strain than those with no children. Moreover, high responsibility for home tasks among employed men and women has been associated with increased ambulatory blood pressure assessed at work, home, and overnight blood pressure, and particularly among women with high job strain (Brisson *et al.* 1999).

Researchers working in the area of work/family conflict in the US have identified areas in which workplaces can become more family-responsive (Glass and Estes 1997, Capowski 1996, Raabe 1990), leading to better outcomes at both the individual and organizational level. Health promotion worksite interventions have in fact been found to be effective especially when health promotion programmes are integrated with occupational health protection programmes (Sorensen *et al.* 1995, Sorensen *et al.* 2002).

In recent years, several large-scale clinical trials have been implemented to modify social networks and social support at an individual level (Berkman *et al.* 2003, Glass *et al.* 2004). By and large these trials have not succeeded in changing health outcomes such as cardiovascular morbidity or mortality nor physical functioning. They have in general had very modest impacts on modifying aspects of social support or network characteristics. If, as many of us believe, social context shapes opportunities for change in terms of social interactions, support, behaviours and ultimately of course for health, then individual-level interventions will never be as powerful as those in which we incorporate contextual elements. How work is organized, the explicit formal policies and benefits in place as well as the less formal culture and set of practices in place among both employers and employees may be one of the most important levers we have to promote health and family functioning, work and community participation and reduce social exclusion and discrimination. We are woefully lacking evidence that specific benefits, practices, or organizational characteristics may be health-promoting. Our hypothesis is that cross-country comparisons can be useful in pointing us in helpful directions and our US/France case study highlights the important differences in social policy that may lead to improvements in population health. The important next steps are to use experimental or quasi-experimental approaches to evaluate the effects of specific policies. Social and economic policies may provide some of our most powerful levers to improve health and well-being by improving the social environment in which we live.

Acknowledgments

This work was supported by The Russel Sage Foundation Program on Inequality and Health and The Workplace, Family, Health, and Well-being Network Funded by NICHD and NIA. The authors express their thanks to EDF-GDF, especially to the services des Etudes Medicales.

References

Bearman P, Moody J, Stovel K (2004). Chains of affection: the structure of adolescent romantic and sexual networks. *American Journal of Sociology*, **110**, 44–91.

Bergmann B (1996). *Saving our children from poverty*. Russell Sage Foundation, New York

Berkman L, Blumenthal J, Burg M and Investigators (2003). Effects of treating depression and low perceived social support on clinical events after myocardial infarction. *Journal of the American Medical Association*, **289**, 3106–16.

Berkman L and Breslow L (1983). *Health and ways of living: the Alameda County Study.* Oxford University Press, New York.

Berkman LF and Glass T (2000). Social integration, social networks, social support and health. In: LF Berkman and I Kawachi (eds) *Social epidemiology*, pp.137–73. Oxford University Press, New York.

Berkman L, Glass T, Brisette I, Seeman T (2000). From social integration to health: Durkheim in the new millennium. *Social Science and Medicine* 51, 843–57.

Berkman L and Kawachi I (eds) (2000). *Social epidemiology.* New York, Oxford University Press.

Berkman L, Melchior M, Chastang J, Niedhammer I, Leclerc A, Goldberg M (2004). Social integration and mortality: a prospective study of French employees of Electricity of France – Gas of France, The GAZEL Cohort. *American Journal of Epidemiology* 159, 167–74.

Berkman L and Syme S (1979). Social networks, host resistance, and mortality: a nine-year follow-up of Alameda County residents. *American Journal of Epidemiology* 109, 186–204.

Blazer D (1982). Social support and mortality in an elderly community population. *American Journal of Epidemiology* 115, 684–94.

Bouvier-Colle M, Magescas J, Hatton F (1985). Causes de décès et jeunes étrangers in France. *Revue d' Epidémiologie et de Santé* 33, 409–16.

Brisson C, Laflamme N, Moisan J, Milot A, Masse B, Vezina M (1999). Effect of family responsibilities and job strain on ambulatory blood pressure among white-collar women. *Psychosomatic Medicine* 61, 205–13.

Capowski G (1996). The job of flex. *Management Review* (**March**), 14–18.

Chevalier A, Leclerc A, Goldberg M (1987). Disparités sociales et professionnelles de la mortalité des travailleurs d'Electricité de France – Gaz de France (in French). *Population* 6, 863–80.

Cohen S (2004). Social relationships and health. *American Psychologist* 59, 676–84.

Committee (2005). Turnout exceeds optimistic predictions: more than 122 million vote, Committee for the Study of the American Electorate.

Cook T (2002). Randomized experiments in educational policy research: a critical examination of the reasons the educational evaluation community has offered for not doing them. *Educational Evaluation and Policy Analysis* 24, 175–99.

Cook T and Campbell D (1979). *Quasi-experimentation: design and analysis issues for field settings.* Houghton Mifflin, Boston, MA.

Dagnet F and Thave S (1996). La population immigrée, le résultat d' une longue histoire. INSEE PREMIERE **458**.

Danzon F, Dressen C, Veil S (1998). *Féminin santé.* Vanves, France, Comite Francais d'Education pour la Santé.

De Carmoy R (1993). Entre intégration et rupture: les adolescentes musulmanes a la recherche de leur identité. *Neuropsychiatrie de l'enfance* 41, 637–43.

Frankenhaeuser M (1989). *Stress, health and job satisfaction.* Stockholm, Sweden, Karolinksa Institute.

Frankenhaeuser M, Lundberg U, Fredrikson M, Melin B, Tuomisto M, Myrsten A (1989). Stress on and off the job as related to sex and occupational status in white-collar workers. *Journal of Organizational Behaviour* 10, 321–46.

Fuhrer R, Shipley MJ, Chastang JF *et al.* (2002). Socioeconomic position, health, and possible explanations: a tale of two cohorts. *American Journal of Public Health*, **92**, 1290–4.

Glass J and Estes S (1997). The family-responsive workplace. *Annual Review of Sociology* **23**, 289–313.

Glass T, Berkman L, Hiltunen E *et al.* (2004). The families in recovery from stroke trial (FIRST): Primary Study Results. *Psychosomatic Medicine* **66**, 889–97.

Granovetter M (1973). The strength of weak ties. *American Journal of Sociology* **78**, 1360–80.

Herpin N and Dechaux JH (2004). Entraide familiale, indépendance économique et sociabilité. *Economie et Statistique* **N 373**, 3–32.

Heymann J (2000). *The widening gap: why American working families are in jeopardy and what can be done about it.* Basic Books, New York.

House J, Robbins C, Metzner H (1982). The association of social relationships and activities with mortality: prospective evidence from the Tecumseh Community Health Study. *American Journal of Epidemiology* **116**, 123–40.

INSEE (2003). Degré de participation associative selon la catégorie socioprofessionnelle. **2005.**

INSEE (2004). La participation électorale selon le niveau de diplôme a age 'contrôle' aux élections de 2004. **2005.**

Kiecolt-Glaser JK, Glaser R, Cacioppo JT (1997). Marital conflict in older adults: endocrinological and immunological correlates. *Psychosomatic Medicine* **59**, 339–49.

Leclerc A, Lert F, Fabien C (1990). Differential mortality: some comparisons between England and Wales, Finland and France, based on inequality measures. *International Journal of Epidemiology* **12**, 1001–10.

Lee S, Colditz G, Berkman L, Chapman Walsh D, Kawachi I (2003). Care-giving and risk of coronary heart disease in US women. *American Journal of Preventive Medicine* **24**, 113–19.

Link B, Phelan J (1995). Social conditions as fundamental causes of disease. *Journal of Health and Social Behavior* (extra issue).

Marsden PV, Friedkin NE (1994). Network studies of social influence. Advances in social network analysis: research in the social and behavioral sciences. In: S Wasserman and J Galaskiewicz (eds) pp. 3–25. Sage, Thousand Oaks, CA.

Melchior M, Goldberg M, Krieger N, Kawachi I, Berkman L (2005). Occupational class, social mobility and cancer incidence among middle-aged men and women: a prospective study of the French Gazel cohort. *Cancer Causes and Control* **16**, 515–240.

OECD (2001). *Panorama de la santé*. Paris, Organisation de Coopération et Développement Economiques.

Orth-Gomer K and Johnson J (1987). Social network interaction and mortality: a six year follow-up study of a random sample of the Swedish population. *Journal of Chronic Disease* **40**, 949–57.

Pan Ke Shon JL (2003). Isolement relationnel et mal-être. INSEE Premiere **N 931**.

Paugam S (1999). Pauvreté, chômage et liens sociaux en Europe. *Données sociales*, INSEE.

Pedersen S (1993). *Family dependence and the origins of the welfare state: Britain and France, 1914–1945.* Cambridge University Press, New York.

Raabe P (1990). The organizational effects of workplace famility policies. *Journal of Family Issues* **11**, 477–81.

Rook K (1992). Detrimental aspects of social relationships: taking stock of an emerging literature. In: HO Veiel and U Baumann (eds) *The meaning and measurement of social support*, pp. 157–69. Hemisphere Publishing Corporation, New York.

Rose G (1992). *The strategy of preventive medicine*. Oxford University Press, New York.

Ross N, Dorling D, Dunn J, Hendricksson G, Glover J, Lynch J (2005). Metropolitan income inequality and working age mortality: a five country analysis using comparable data. *Journal of Urban Health* **82**, 101–10.

Schulz R and Beach S (1999). Care-giving as a risk factor for mortality. *Journal of the American Medical Association* **282**, 2215–19.

Shon PK (1999). Vivre seul, sentiment de solitude et isolement relationnel. INSEE Premiere **678**, 1–3.

Sorensen G, Himmelstein J, Hunt M *et al.* (1995). A model for worksite cancer prevention: Integration of health protection and health promotion in the WellWorks project. *American Journal of Health Promotion* **10**, 55–62.

Sorensen G, Stoddard A, LaMontagne A *et al.* (2002). A comprehensive worksite cancer prevention intervention: behavior change results from a randomized controlled trial in manufacturing worksites (United States). *Cancer Causes and Control* **13**, 493–502.

Sugisawa H, Liang J, Liu X (1994). Social networks, social support and mortality among older people in Japan. *Journal of Gerontology* **49**, S3–13.

Thave S (2000). L'emploi des immigrés en 1999. INSEE Premiere N 717.

Wilkinson R (2005). *The impact of inequality: how to make sick societies healthier*. The New Press, London.

Zins M, Gueguen A, Nakache J *et al.* (2003). Do lifestyle factors explain social health inequalities? A ten year follow-up of the mortality of men of the French GAZEL cohort. XXI Annual Scientific Conference of the Spanish Epidemiology Society/European Epidemiology Federation, Toledo, Spain.

Chapter 4

Socio-economic position and health

The role of work and employment

Johannes Siegrist and Töres Theorell

Introduction

Work and employment are of critical importance for health. Exposure to adverse working conditions contributes to the burden of disease in a variety of ways. Physical and chemical hazards, physically demanding work, long or irregular working hours, shiftwork, health-adverse posture, extended sedentary work and a broad range of psychological and social stressors at work were shown to adversely affect the health of working people. In all these instances exposure time is relevant as the risk of disease increases over time, often in a dose-response relationship.

For a large part of the population in early, middle, and early old adulthood, work has primary significance as it is normally a prerequisite for a regular income which in turn determines a wide range of life chances. Moreover, work provides opportunities of personal performance, learning and achievement by confronting people with recurrent challenges and demands. It is mainly through work and employment that social status in adulthood is acquired and that a core social identity outside the family is developed and maintained. Therefore, in addition to the quality of work, employment conditions in terms of security, continuity and promotion prospects are important for health and well-being. This has been documented by a large body of research on health-adverse effects of unemployment, precarious work, forced downward mobility and involuntary early exit from the labour market (see below).

The quality of work and employment is socially graded, with individuals having low educational attainments and qualifications being confined to less favourable jobs and those with higher qualifications being offered better jobs. As many highly prevalent diseases in current societies follow a social gradient, leaving those in lower socio-economic positions in worse health, the question arises to what extent and by which mechanisms work and employment contribute to the development of social inequalities in adult health. The importance of this question is further emphasized by the fact that after the first years of childhood, midlife is the time when social differences in morbidity and mortality are most pronounced.

This chapter sets out to explore the role of work and employment in explaining social inequalities in health by focusing on material and psychosocial dimensions of an adverse work environment. First, two influential theoretical models – demand–control and effort–reward – are discussed that aim at identifying 'toxic' components within the complexities of stressful working conditions and empirical evidence supporting their role in the development of ill health and disease is presented. Second, the suitability of these models for tackling new challenges of the currently witnessed globalization and transformation of work and employment is analysed. Following this, we discuss two different aspects of the role of work in explaining unequal health: (a) pathways into paid work and (b) adversity at work as a determinant of socially graded morbidity and mortality. In this latter approach we distinguish between mediation and effect modification. Finally, policy implications of new knowledge on links between work and social inequalities in health are addressed.

Theoretical models and empirical evidence

Demand–control and effort–reward imbalance

Occupational health research has long been concerned with the material dimensions of health-adverse work, in particular physical and chemical hazards and physically strenuous jobs. While these conditions are causally related to diseases occurring within specific occupations (the occupational diseases), they are of less importance in explaining health inequalities according to occupational standing in a variety of different occupations and professions. Today, fewer jobs are defined by physical demands and more by mental and emotional demands. Computer-based information processing is becoming a part of a growing number of job profiles, and employment in the service sector continues to rise. As a result, psychological and social stressors are becoming more prevalent, and their contribution to health and well-being at work is likely to parallel or even outweigh the contribution of more traditional occupational stressors.

An adverse psychosocial environment at work cannot be identified by direct physical or chemical measurements. Theoretical concepts are needed to delineate particular stressful job characteristics so that they can be identified at a level of generalization that allows for their use in a wide range of different occupations. These concepts are then translated into measures with the help of social science research methods (standardized questionnaires, observation techniques etc.) that meet the criteria of adequate reliability and validity of data collection. While several concepts of an adverse psychosocial work environment have been developed (Cooper 1998, Perrewe and Ganster 2002), two models have received special attention in recent years: the demand–control model and the effort–reward imbalance model.

The demand–control model was introduced by Karasek (1979) and further developed by Karasek and Theorell (1990). It posits that stressful experience at work results from a distinct job task profile defined by two dimensions, the psychological demands put on the working person and the degree of control available to the person to perform the required tasks. Jobs defined by high demands and low control are stressful because they limit the individual's autonomy and sense of control while generating continued pressure (high job strain). Under these conditions, excessive arousal of the autonomic nervous system is expected to occur (catabolic state) that is not compensated by a relaxation response following the experience of control and mastery (anabolic state).

Importantly, a low level of control or decision latitude manifests itself in two ways, first as lack of decision authority over one's tasks, and second as a low level of skill utilization, as evidenced by monotonous, repetitive work. While task profiles defined by low decision latitude in combination with low demands too may adversely affect health – although to a lesser extent than 'high strain jobs' – 'active jobs' are expected to be health-protective or even health-promoting. Such jobs are defined by challenging demands that go along with a high degree of decision authority and learning opportunities. Active jobs enable individuals to experience positive stimulation, success and self efficacy. Under these conditions, autonomic arousal is balanced by anabolic states of relaxation. It is obvious that some of the traditional high strain jobs are found in mass industry, especially under conditions of piece work and machine paced assembly line work. Nevertheless, a variety of high demand–low control task profiles were identified in administrative jobs dealing with information processing and, even more so, in the service sector.

A third dimension, social support at work, was added to the original formulation. Karasek (1979) and Karasek and Theorell (1990) introduced the demand/control/support model where highest strain is expected to occur in jobs that are characterized by high demand, low control and low social support at work or social isolation (iso-strain jobs). Conversely, available social support at work may mitigate the amount of stress in people confined to high strain jobs. The support dimension was tested and discussed in more detail for the first time by Johnson and Hall (1990).

As is the case with most theoretical concepts, they tend to highlight particular aspects of the complex reality at the expense of other aspects that are considered as being of minor importance. However, some of the neglected aspects may be relevant to the topic under study. This is the reason for emerging complementary models. One such complementary model, termed effort–reward imbalance, is concerned with stressful features of the work contract (Siegrist *et al.* 1986, Siegrist 1996). This model builds on the notion of social reciprocity, a fundamental principle rooted in an evolutionary old grammar of interpersonal exchange. Social reciprocity lies at the core of the employment (or work) contract which defines distinct obligations or tasks to be performed in exchange with adequate rewards. These rewards include money, esteem and career opportunities, including job security. Contractual reciprocity operates through norms of return expectancy, where efforts spent by employees are reciprocated by equitable rewards from employers. The effort–reward imbalance model claims that lack of reciprocity occurs frequently under specific conditions (see below) and that failed reciprocity in terms of high cost and low gain elicits strong negative emotions with a special propensity to sustained autonomic and neuroendocrine activation and their adverse long-term consequences for health. According to the theory, contractual non-reciprocity is expected if one or several of the following conditions are given: dependency, strategic choice, and overcommitment.

Dependency reflects the structural constraints observed in certain types of employment contracts, especially so in unskilled or semi-skilled workers, in elderly employees, in employees with restricted mobility or limited work ability, and in workers with short-term contracts. In all these instances, incentives of paying non-equitable rewards are high for employers, while the risks of rejecting an unfair contractual transaction by employees are low. The reason for this asymmetrical exchange is best described by one of the founders of economic theory, John Stuart Mill

> The really exhausting and the really repulsive labours, instead of being better paid than others, are almost invariably paid the worst of all, because performed by those who have no choice. The inequalities of wages are generally in an opposite direction to the equitable principle of compensation. (Mill 1848/1962, p. 383)

Non-symmetrical contractual exchange due to lack of alternative choice in the labour market is relatively frequent in modern economies that are characterized by a globalized labour market, mergers and organizational downsizing, rapid technological change, and a high level of job instability.

Strategic choice is a second condition of non-symmetrical exchange. Here, people accept high cost/low gain conditions of their employment for a certain time, often without being forced to do so, because they tend to improve their chances of career promotion and related rewards at a later stage. This pattern is frequently observed in early stages of professional careers and in jobs that are characterized by heavy competition. As anticipatory investments are made on the basis of insecure return expectancy, the risk of failed success after long-lasting efforts is considerable. In fact, negative life events resulting from overt contract violation were shown to exert particularly harmful effects on people's well-being and health (Siegrist 1984).

Third, there are psychological reasons for a recurrent mismatch between efforts and rewards at work. People characterized by a motivational pattern of excessive work-related *overcommitment* may strive towards continuously high achievement because of their underlying need for approval and esteem at work. Although these excessive efforts are often not met by adequate rewards, overcommitted people tend to maintain their level of involvement. There is reason to believe that this motivational style affects how demands are appraised. Perceptual distortion prevents overcommitted people from accurately assessing cost–gain relations. As a consequence, they underestimate the demands, and overestimate their own coping resources while not being aware of their own contribution to non-reciprocal exchange. Work-related overcommitment is elicited and reinforced by a variety of job environments, and is often experienced as self-rewarding over a period of years in occupational trajectories. However, in the long run, overcommitted people are susceptible to exhaustion and adaptive breakdown (see below).

In summary, the model of effort–reward imbalance at work maintains that non-symmetric contractual exchange is frequent under these structural and personal conditions, and that people experiencing dependency, strategic choice or overcommitment, either separately or in combination, are at elevated risk of suffering from stress-related disorders.

As mentioned, the two models complement each other by focusing on toxic components of job task profiles and employment contracts respectively. Low control and low reward are assumed to be equally stressful experiences in the context of effortful work. They both elicit negative emotions that are paralleled by excessive activation of the autonomic nervous system. It is therefore likely that simultaneously experienced low control and low reward in demanding jobs may increase the probability of ill health above and beyond the risk associated with separate exposure to these conditions.

Empirical evidence

Epidemiological studies

Both models have been extensively tested using a variety of study designs: prospective observational studies, case-control and cross-sectional investigations, laboratory experiments, 'naturalistic' studies with ambulatory monitoring techniques, and intervention studies. Several reviews are currently available that document the state of the art (Belkic *et al.* 2004, Marmot *et al.* 2002, Tsutsumi and Kawakami 2004, van Vegchel *et al.* 2005). The prospective epidemiological observational study is considered a gold standard approach in this field because of its temporal sequence (exposure assessment precedes disease onset), its sample size (based on statistical power calculation and allowing for adjustment for confounding variables in multivariate analysis) and the quantification of subsequent disease risk following exposure (odds ratio of disease in exposed vs. non-exposed individuals). Therefore, we provide a short summary of the main findings based on prospective studies. However, given the variety of stress-related disorders of interest and the relative paucity of prospective investigations of incident diseases other than cardiovascular disease, we include selected findings from other types of studies.

At present, more than 20 reports derived from prospective studies of associations between work stress and cardiovascular disease are available, with a majority testing the job strain model. In six of these reports, the effort–reward imbalance model was investigated, partly in comparison with the demand–control model. Although measures were not fully comparable across these studies, the majority of findings support either the full theoretical models or their main components (Belkic *et al.* 2004, Marmot *et al.* 2002, van Vegchel *et al.* 2005). Odds ratios or hazard ratios vary considerably across the studies, but, overall, a twofold elevated risk is observed among individuals with high work stress in terms of 'job strain' or effort–reward imbalance, compared to non-exposed individuals. Findings are more consistent in men than in women, and more consistent in middle-aged as compared to early-old-aged populations. The observation period in these studies varies from one to 25 years, with a mean eight years.

For several reasons, the Valmet study of 812 employees of a metalworking company in Finland provides a particularly instructive case of this type of investigations. The study covers a mean observation period of 25.6 years, it contains validated measures of both work stress models, and information on outcome, cardiovascular mortality, was obtained from the national mortality register. Moreover, data on socio-economic conditions were collected with reference to two stages of the cohort's life course, early childhood (father's occupational group, among others) and early adulthood (salary at study onset, among others). As can be seen from Figure 4.1, hazard ratios for cardiovascular mortality by levels of work stress remained fairly stable when adjustments for these two sets of socio-economic covariates were made (Brunner *et al.* 2004).

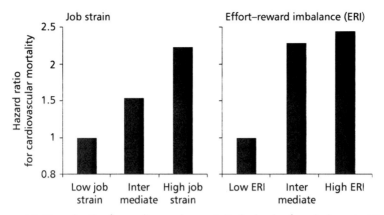

Figure 4.1 Hazard ratios for cardiovascular mortality by levels of work characteristics in the Valmet study adjusted for age, sex and father's occupational group; similar results when models are adjusted for alternative measures of socioeconomic position (height, education, own occupational group, income at baseline). (Based on Brunner et al. (2004).

Yet several studies found no association between work stress and cardiovascular disease. It has been argued that in some of these studies, the sample was relatively old (Reed et al. 1989, Suadicani et al. 1993, Eaker et al. 2004) or biased in terms of health selection (Hlatky et al. 1995). Whether improvements in measuring the models or new ways of combining or refining them may lead to further progress remains to be seen.

Affective disorders, incident type 2 diabetes and alcohol dependence were additional health outcomes in prospective studies testing the two work stress models. Relatively consistent findings were reported for either model with regard to depression (Stansfeld et al. 1999) although the majority of studies confirming these associations are cross-sectional investigations (Niedhammer et al. 1998, Pikhart et al. 2004, Tsutsumi et al. 2001, Larisch et al. 2003). Incident type 2 diabetes and alcohol dependence were prospectively associated with effort–reward imbalance at work in men, but not in women (Head et al. 2004, Kumari et al. 2004). The odds ratios in these reports based on the British Whitehall II study were 1.6 and 1.9 respectively.

In terms of economic impact of work-related burden of disease, musculoskeletal disorders and sick leave are of primary importance. Several cross-sectional (Joksimovic et al. 2002, Vingård et al. 2000, Wigaeus et al. 2001) and prospective studies (Hemingway et al. 1997, Kaila-Kangas et al. 2004, Hoogendoorn et al. 2002) explored associations of work stress with musculoskeletal disorders, obtaining mixed results. One conclusion from these findings is that it is difficult to disentangle the effects of psychosocial and physical strain as these two are often highly correlated.

Until recently, sick leave has been studied more intensively with respect to the demand–control model. Several large-scale investigations found that people working in high demand/low control jobs are at elevated risk of sickness absence. This was the case for the JACE study in Belgium (Moreau *et al.* 2004), the Whitehall II study in the United Kingdom (North *et al.* 1996), and a Swedish study (Oxenstierna *et al.* 2005). In this latter investigation, low decision authority was a consistent predictor of long spells of sick leave (more than sixty days). In addition, those who reported poor social support from work colleagues had an increased risk of long-term sickness absence. New prospective evidence from a large-scale study in Finland indicates that effort–reward imbalance at work predicts sickness absence as well as job strain (Ala-Mursula *et al.* 2005). However, as will be shown below, when studying work-related determinants of sick leave, a broader approach is needed where work stress is linked to macroeconomic changes (see below).

In summary, an extended body of evidence indicates that in a majority of studies an adverse psychosocial work environment in terms of job strain and/or effort–reward imbalance is associated with poor health, as measured by a variety of objective and subjective parameters. Knowledge on this association is relatively most advanced in case of cardiovascular risk and disease where important psychobiological processes underlying the observed statistical association have been elucidated in the recent past (Stansfeld and Marmot 2002, see also chapter 5 in this volume).

Naturalistic studies

One such important psychobiological process concerns the activation of the hypothalamic–pituitary–adrenocortical stress axis that plays a crucial role in mediating signals from the central nervous system to the periphery of the organism, in particular in the regulation of energy mobilization (see chapter 5 and 6, in this volume). As cortisol excretion follows a diurnal pattern it is mandatory to interpret variation in hormonal release in the context of circadian rhythm. To date, cortisol excretion can be assessed in urine, blood serum and saliva. Saliva cortisol is easily collected, which makes it possible to record circadian rhythms (Kirschbaum and Hellhammer 1999). In general, high levels of energy correspond to high concentrations of this hormone. Under normal conditions, this is reflected in elevated levels of morning cortisol and reduced levels in the evening. However, disturbed feedback regulation of this stress axis following extensive, prolonged stress-related activation was shown to result in a reduced ability of down-regulating hormonal release as well as in a reduced ability to respond to external challenges. As these conditions were observed with higher prevalence in individuals who suffer from stress-related disorders (Rosmond and Bjorntorp 2000, Cleary 2000), it is of interest to explore whether they also parallel exposure to stressful working conditions.

So far, research on the association between cortisol secretion and work stress has produced mixed results (see chapter 5 and 6 in this volume). It seems that introducing person characteristics into the analysis may add to the explanatory power of respective studies (Steptoe *et al.* 2000, 2004). A further refinement concerns the analysis of effects of exposure time. As it was suggested that prolonged exposure to stressful work may reduce hormonal responsiveness several studies did show reduced rather than heightened cortisol responses following stressful exposure (Fujiwara *et al.* 2004, Siegrist *et al.* 1997, chapter 6 in this volume).

On the other hand, analysis of cortisol excretion may be differentiated according to responsiveness status. This means that individuals with blunted responsiveness during the work day should be analysed separately from individuals who exhibit a pattern of diurnal responsiveness. In one recent Swedish study this differentiation was analysed.

Figures 4.2a and b show mean saliva cortisol concentration in different groups of working women in the PART study (an epidemiological study of mental health in randomly selected men and women in Stockholm). Figure 4.2 shows the results from the total sample of working women (altogether n = 348) since the number of men was smaller and findings for them were non-significant. Ages varied between 20 and 64, but age had no influence on saliva cortisol. The saliva cortisol concentration was significantly lower in the low strain group than in the other groups half an hour after awakening. In the afternoon and evening there were no differences between the demand–control categories. The analysis of variance was not significant for the whole model when all occasions and all groups were tested in a joint model despite the differences between the groups half an hour after awakening. The three groups with low control, high demand or the combination were statistically indistinguishable.

An analysis was also performed in which participants with either consistently high cortisol which did not decrease at bedtime ('evening high'), or consistently low cortisol which did not rise in the morning ('flat low'), were excluded from the analysis. The rationale behind this was that the regulatory system should be preserved. If not, no relationship between working conditions and cortisol concentration can be predicted. These results for female participants are shown in Figure 4.2b. The whole statistical model in the analysis of variance in this case was clearly significant both with regard to cortisol concentration in general and with regard to interaction between occasion

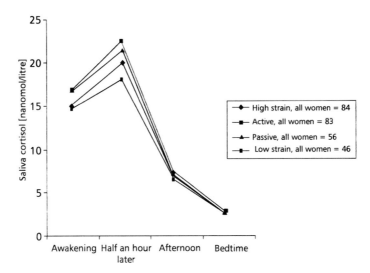

Figure 4.2(a) Saliva cortisol in relation to demand–control group and time of day, all working PART women.

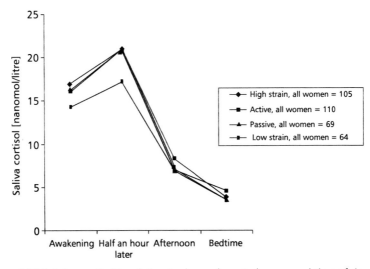

Figure 4.2(b) Saliva cortisol in relation to demand–control group and time of day. Working women in PART after exclusion of high and flat curves.

and group (p = 0.02 in both cases). Again the low strain group (n = 46) had clearly lower means than the other groups, and again the high strain (n = 84), 'active' (n = 83) and 'passive' (n = 56) groups could not be differentiated from one another. The more restricted analysis thus allows us to make a safer conclusion than the analysis of the total group although both analyses point in the same direction. Medication made no difference to this conclusion (Alderling *et al.* 2005). The main finding is that in women the low strain category had lower morning saliva cortisol than the others and that this was particularly clear in the restricted analysis (Alderling *et al.* 2005). Studies of cortisol regulation in subjects with job strain and imbalance between effort and reward have not shown a consistent picture. However, disturbed regulation has been observed in several studies.

Apart from hormonal measures several studies investigated associations of work stress with cardiovascular activity (heart rate, heart rate variability, elevated blood pressure). In general, marked changes in the expected direction were observed (Collins *et al.* 2004, Landsbergis *et al.* 2003, Rau *et al.* 2001, Steptoe and Willemsen 2004, Theorell *et al.* 1988, Vrijkotte *et al.* 2000), although some studies found effects with single components of the two models only or with objective as opposed to subjective measures of stressful work.

Blood pressure regulation has been studied extensively in relation to decision latitude and job strain. The study of working men in New York City (Landsbergis *et al.* 2003) has shown consistent relationships between a high life exposure to job strain and high systolic blood pressure during continuous blood pressure recordings in prospective analyses. They also found strong cross-sectional associations between job strain and both systolic and diastolic blood pressure (Schnall *et al.* 2000).

For many years it was believed that there is no relationship between blood pressure measured in the conventional way (in the doctor's office) and job strain described as a stable job characteristic. Two prospective population studies have recently shown that job strain does predict incident hypertension even when other factors have been adjusted. The first one was the CARDIA study in the USA (Markovitz *et al.* 2004) which followed 3200 employed initially healthy normotensive subjects aged 20 to 32 from 1987–1988 for 8 years. Subjects who had had increased job strain were more likely than others to have developed hypertension. The other study is a Canadian population study (Brisson *et al.* 2004). The evidence is growing that psychosocial factors may contribute to elevated plasma fibrinogen, an indicator of inflammatory activity and increased coagulation (see Theorell 2002 and chapter 5 this volume). Accordingly adverse long-lasting psychosocial conditions may induce bodily states that increase the vulnerability to illness. Enhanced coagulation and increased inflammatory activity could both be regarded as phenomena that accompany energy mobilization. Interleukin-6 concentration in serum has been studied in relation to the demand control model in a Swedish study

(Theorell *et al.* 2000). In this study, low decision latitude was associated with high serum interleukin-6 in men, but not in women.

There is much less evidence showing decreased anabolic/regenerative activity during periods of job strain and/or imbalance between effort and reward. Regenerative activity is reflected in the serum concentration of testosterone (men), oestrogen (women) and their joint precursor DHEA-s. A longitudinal study of variations in job strain in men showed that periods of high job strain were associated with lowered serum concentration of testosterone (Theorell *et al.* 1991). Hansen *et al.* (2003) studied metabolic and endocrine concomitants of repetitive work (sewing machine operators) which was shown to be associated with increased glycated hemoglobin (an indicator of long term energy mobilization) as well as lowered serum concentration of DHEA-s and free testosterone. A one-year follow-up study in the late 1990s in Sweden (Hertting and Theorell 2002) showed that female health care staff had a lowered serum concentration of oestradiol after having been exposed to and adjusted to recurrent organizational downsizing. Yet current evidence on impact of work stress on regeneration is much weaker than is the case with energy mobilization.

In summary, physiological and biochemical studies provide important scientific support of epidemiological evidence derived from large-scale prospective and cross-sectional studies on the association of work stress with reduced health.

Macroeconomic contexts of work stress and health

The components of both work stress models reflect job conditions that are directly influenced by macroeconomic developments. In particular, with the advent of economic globalization in combination with progress in information technology, competition between companies and pressure towards an increase of return on investment have been growing over the past two decades. As a consequence, work pressure increased considerably in several private sectors of national economies, but also in public sectors, due to financial cuts in public expenditures (Eurostat 2004). Another consequence of economic globalization concerns the segmentation of the labour market and a related increase in income inequality. On the one hand, there is a well-trained, skilled and flexible workforce with a high level of job satisfaction, fair promotion prospects and adequate earnings. On the other hand, a large part of the workforce in advanced societies suffers from job insecurity, low wages and salaries, and a low level of control of work schedules and job conditions. Less qualified, less mobile and older workers are more likely to belong to the latter segment (Benach *et al.* 2002).

Several large scale investigations recently explored health–adverse consequences of these economic developments in combination with work-related stress. Convincing evidence is available from studies on adverse health effects produced by organizational downsizing indicating that 'survivors' of these stressful transitions are at increased risk, in addition to those who are laid off. Elevated levels of sickness absence (Kivimäki et al. 2001, Westerlund et al. 2004a) and even mortality (Vahtera et al. 2004) were reported, among others.

However, the separate and combined effects of macrostructural (downsizing) and microstructural (stressful everyday work) conditions were explored only recently in a study conducted in an 0.1 per cent random sample of the German workforce (Dragano et al. 2005). Associations of the separate and combined effects of organizational downsizing and work stress, as measured by effort–reward imbalance, on poor self-rated health (number of work-related symptoms) were analysed. Compared with the reference group, employees who were simultaneously exposed to downsizing and effort–reward imbalance exhibited odds ratios of work-related symptoms that were by far higher than those with single exposures. Single exposures, too, were associated with significantly reduced health (Dragano et al. 2005). During the past 15 years there have been pronounced work life changes going on in several European countries. Accordingly it has become important to explore the extent to which psychosocial working conditions interact with structural changes in generating worsened employee health and possibly changes in social inequality in health.

Sweden is an interesting case in this context. During the 1990s Sweden went through a pronounced financial crisis which resulted in markedly increased unemployment rates. Some economic recovery took place during the latter part of the decade, at the expense of increasing demands and decreasing decision authority, most pronounced in the public sector of employment (Theorell 2004). In the period of 1997 to 2001, a sharp increase of long-term sick leave was observed in the public employment sector, particularly among women (Westerlund et al. 2004a). The biennial national Swedish Work Environment survey offered an opportunity to analyse the impact of expanding and shrinking organizations on sickness absence and hospital admissions in a prospective design. Long-term ($\geq$ 90 days) medically certified sickness absence and hospital admissions for specified diagnoses (cardiovascular, musculoskeletal, gastrointestinal and psychiatric) during 1997 to 1999 were related to changes in the composition of the organizations' workforce in previous years (1991 to 1996) in an interesting way. In general elevated odds ratios of long-term sickness absence and hospitalization were found in employees who were working in organizations with large personnel expansion compared to those working in stable organizations (Westerlund *et al.* 2004a). In the same comparison with stable organizations, slow moderate expansion of personnel, on the other hand, was associated with reduced hospitalization risk. It is obvious that slow expansion could be regarded as a 'healthy' sign whereas rapid pronounced expansion may be associated with tensions. This was verified when work environment descriptions of these employees were compared to those in stable organizations: a large expansion of personnel was associated with a low decision authority whereas a moderate expansion was associated with good social support and good decision authority. These findings were particularly clear for long-term sickness absence among women in the public sector. Rapid expansion in the public sector has often been due to centralization of units during this period. In interviews with managers in the different work sites included in the WOLF study Westerlund *et al.* (2004b) showed that they could be divided into stable and changing worksites. Employees in stable worksites had less job strain and lower cardiovascular risk than other employees. Rapid expansion of personnel was also prevalent in the private sector of the Swedish economy, but was less consistently associated with long-term sickness absence. This finding could be explained in part by 'sickness presenteeism' (Aronsson *et al.* 2000), a pattern of repressed need of recovery and repressed need of being treated while ill. This was also illustrated in another study which showed that a proxy measure of extrinsic imbalance between effort and reward was in general associated with a prospectively recorded elevation of long-term sickness absence incidence (Jeding *et al.* 2006), the exception being men in the private sector. In this group no association was found between effort–reward imbalance and long-term sick leave despite pronounced elevation of psychosomatic symptom prevalence. Sickness presenteeism was found to be relatively frequent in highly competitive private organizations (Aronsson *et al.* 2000). A further Swedish study analysed the association of expanding or shrinking organizations with 'absenteeism' or 'presenteeism' in a group of employees who were already at risk of developing cardiovascular disease (Theorell *et al.* 2003). Subjects were 5720 employees aged 18 to 65 in the WOLF study (a prospective study of biological and psychosocial cardiovascular risk factors in working men and women in the Stockholm area during the years 1992–1995). From a medical examination a cardiovascular risk score was calculated for each participant. The WOLF study base was linked to national registers of economic and administrative activities in work sites. Work sites with downsizing (at least 8 per cent decrease from one year to the next), stable number of staff (changes less than 8 per cent decrease or 8 per cent increase) and expansion ($>$ 8 per cent increase) were identified. Sick leave spells lasting for at least 15 days during the calendar year following the downsizing/expansion were identified through individual linkage with the national insurance register.

Interestingly, among women it was found that sickness absence during the year following both downsizing and expansion was decreased compared to the group of women employed in stable work sites. This may again reflect some pressure towards 'sickness presenteeism' because the trend was particularly pronounced among women with an elevated cardiovascular risk score (Theorell *et al.* 2003).

These findings illustrate the importance of including structural changes of labour market and work, in particular downsizing and continued rapid expansion, into research on work stress and health.

Social inequalities, work and health

So far, we demonstrated that an adverse work environment as defined by the demand–control and the effort–reward imbalance models reduces the health and well being of exposed people and that these effects are magnified by macro-economic constraints resulting in work intensification and increased threats to occupational control and reward. As mentioned at the beginning of this chapter, adversity at work is socially graded, leaving those with low qualification, the unskilled and semi-skilled segments of the workforce, at highest risk of precarious employment and job loss. There is robust evidence that at least core components of the two work stress models, low decision latitude and low reward (especially salary, promotion prospects and job security) follow a social gradient (Bosma *et al.* 1998, Brunner *et al.* 2004, Niedhammer *et al.* 2000). The situation is less consistent with regard to the full models as high demands, high extrinsic and intrinsic effort at work are often more prevalent in higher status groups (Karasek and Theorell 1990, Siegrist *et al.* 2004).

Here, the question arises how current knowledge on the health burden of work-related stress can improve our understanding of the social gradient of morbidity and mortality in midlife and early old age. In the following para-graphs, two complementary answers to this question are given by considering pathways into paid work and by analysing mediation and effect modification in associations between socio-economic position, work stress and health.

Pathways into paid work

Critics of the field of research on psychosocial stress at work and health have argued that observed work stress effects may be attributable to confounding with early childhood adversity that predisposes people to being selected into more stressful jobs in adult life (Macleod *et al.* 2001). It is therefore important to analyse available evidence that supports or contradicts this argument. First, it was clearly shown that children with low status parental background have a lower probability of experiencing upward mobility later on as compared to children with middle class social background (see chapter 2 in this volume). They are thus more likely to end up in semi-skilled or unskilled jobs associated with elevated health risks. Yet it is not clear how strong this effect may be. For instance, in a large British study, it was recently demonstrated that intelligence test scores in childhood are associated with social mobility in an uniform pattern, regardless of parental socio-economic position: the higher the score, the higher the probability of being upwardly mobile (Nettle 2003). Thus, it is unlikely that material deprivation in childhood per se predicts an unfavourable occupational trajectory later on, especially so as the association of parental social background with intelligence is generally lower than the association of adult socio-economic position with intelligence. Second, even if a selection effect operates in producing unequal adult health, it remains to be seen how strong this effect is if compared to the direct effect produced by exposure to an adverse work environment. Several studies have answered this question. In the Valmet study mentioned above, adjustment for childhood socio-economic conditions did not reduce the strength of the association of work stress with cardiovascular mortality (Brunner *et al.* 2004). Similarly, the Whitehall II study found that adult socio-economic position was a more important predictor of morbidity attributable to coronary disease, depression and chronic bronchitis than measures of social status earlier in life (Marmot *et al.* 2001), indicating that living and working conditions associated with adult social status are of primary importance in this regard. A recent longitudinal study from France confirms this finding as an unfavourable occupational trajectory in adulthood predicts mortality more strongly than deprived early life circumstances (Melchior *et al.* 2006). Finally, the association of work stress in terms of effort–reward imbalance and job strain, with early atherosclerosis (as assessed by ultrasound carotid intima media thickness) remained substantial and statistically significant after adjusting for a number of relevant early childhood factors (Kivimäki *et al.* 2006).

In summary, several studies from different countries using different health indicators resulted in the same conclusion: while early life is clearly important for adult health, the effects attributable to exposure to adversity at work in adult life are consistently stronger than these former effects. This conclusion supports the relevance of a life course perspective in studying social inequalities in health.

Mediation and effect modification

If work stress is more prevalent in lower socio-economic groups and if both work stress and low social status are associated with reduced health, it is tempting to conclude that work stress mediates the association of socio-economic status with health. In fact, some evidence in support of the mediation hypothesis has been found. In the Whitehall II study, low control at work was independently associated with incident coronary disease and with low socio-economic status (Marmot *et al.* 1997). In multivariate analysis, low control in the workplace accounted for about half the social gradient of coronary heart disease as the odds ratio of coronary disease in the low employment group was reduced from about 1.4 to about 1.2 after respective adjustment. Importantly, the relation between low control and coronary disease was not removed by adjusting for socio-economic position (Marmot *et al.* 1997; see also Chapter 7 in this volume). Similar findings were obtained in a case-control study of coronary patients in the Czech republic (Bobak *et al.* 1998).

Mediation is important, but it is not the only way that a variable that predicts disease incidence in populations may contribute towards explaining the association of socio-economic status with morbidity and mortality. The effect modification hypothesis posits that susceptibility to an exposure (such as work stress) is higher among lower status compared to higher status people and, therefore, that among people with lower socio-economic status, the effect size produced by the exposure is higher.

The effect modification hypothesis was tested in several studies that documented a stronger effect of high demand and low control at work, or of high effort and low reward at work, on risk of coronary disease incidence in lower status groups (Johnson and Hall 1988, Hallqvist *et al.* 1998, Kuper *et al.* 2002). For instance, Kuper *et al.* (2002) analysed the association of effort–reward imbalance to coronary disease incidence (quartiles of the effort–reward ratio) in an 11 year follow-up period in the Whitehall II study. While they found an increased disease risk in the upper quartile of scores in the effort–reward ratio within the total study population, this effect was relatively strongest in the lowest employment group, especially so for fatal and non-fatal acute myocardial infarction (see Figure 4.3).

By reducing health and well-being, continued stressful experience at work compromises the work ability of people. Most important among the occupational characteristics that predict early retirement are those that show a high prevalence in lower socio-economic status groups: jobs with a low degree of substantive complexity, repetitive tasks, jobs with low level of control and autonomy at work and with heavy physical demands. These jobs are often

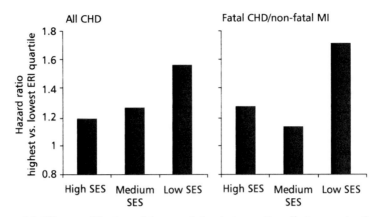

Figure 4.3 Effect modification of the association between the effort–reward ratio and coronary heart disease by employment grade (Whitehall II-Study; 11 year follow-up, N = 10,308 male and female civil servants). Based on Kuper *et al.* (2002).

associated with exposure to noise and other physical or chemical stressors, uncomfortable working positions and elevated risk of injury. More recently, the two models of psychosocial stress at work were explicitly tested with regard to early retirement. In a large Norwegian sample, strong links were found between high demand/low control jobs and both types of early exit from work, disability-related and non-disability-related early retirement among men, but not among women (Blekesaune and Solem 2005). High effort/low reward conditions were associated with risk of disability-related early retirement in a recent German case-control study with census data from a wide variety of occupations (N. Dragano, personal communication).

The increased health burden of low socio-economic position, as defined by occupational status and associated adverse working conditions, is still visible decades after exit from work. This impressive finding was obtained from the first Whitehall Study of British civil servants, of men aged 40 to 69 when first studied. Thirty years later, at re-survey, the median age of respondents was 77 years (range 67–97). Men were classified according to their grade of employment at entry to the study. Social gradients in four different measures of health and functioning were found three decades later. Overall, a doubling of risk between high grade and low grade civil servants was observed for mental health and disability, and a threefold elevated risk was observed for general health and physical performance (Breeze *et al.* 2001). Taken together, evidence indicates that social inequalities in midlife and in older age are strongly influenced by adverse circumstances of work and employment. Therefore, policy implications of this new knowledge need to be addressed.

Policy implications

Improving the quality of work and employment is a target that can be tackled at several levels. International and national regulations and policies are far-reaching approaches. It is encouraging to see a growing interest among organizations such as the European Commission, the World Health Organization, and the International Labour Organization, to deal with measures of reducing work-related stress. National policies vary quite substantially in this regard, depending on level of economic development, welfare regime and political preferences (see Chapter 9 and 10 in this volume). With the advent of economic globalization, national policies of work-related health and safety measures and of fair employment are increasingly challenged by options of labour force mobility and flexibility and of capital flow across boundaries that are available to multinational private organizations and companies. These options threaten national standards and undermine important progress that has been achieved by trade unions (Landsbergis 2003).

Single companies (especially medium- and large-scale organizations) are probably the most effective target of intervention approaches. In this chapter we have argued that two theoretical models hold particular promise in explaining work-related disease, the demand–control and effort–reward imbalance models. The conditions identified by these models provide a framework in which to understand and to modify the contribution of psychosocial factors at work to the development of disease.

The conceptual differences between the models have direct implications for the design of intervention measures to improve health. Whereas the emphasis of the demand–control model is on change of the task structure (such as job enlargement, job enrichment and increasing the amount of support within the job etc.) the focus of the effort–reward imbalance model is on contractual fairness in terms of reciprocity between cost and gain. This latter model offers measures at three levels, the individual level (e.g. reduction of overcommitment), the interpersonal level (e.g. improvement of leadership, of providing esteem reward), and the structural level (e.g. compensatory wage systems, models of gain sharing, and strengthening of non-monetary gratifications). Both models stress the need for better opportunities of job training, of learning new skills and of increasing job security. In addition to general measures, more specific measures can be tailored for special risk groups at work, most importantly elderly workers.

As illustrated below, several intervention studies were conducted along these lines. Yet, in general, it has been difficult to evaluate direct health effects. One of the main reasons for these difficulties concerns a constantly changing labour market and rapid organizational changes, e.g. due to mergers, outsourcing or other major structural changes. Such changes may make it impossible to interpret the intervention process and its expected outcomes. However, particularly in the Scandinavian setting, evaluations of health effects of organizational changes aiming at improved worker participation have been made (for a summary, see Wahlstedt 2001).

For instance, the effort–reward imbalance model has been the basis of an intervention for bus drivers (Kompier *et al.* 2002). With a main focus on the job demand–control model, the Stockholm group has performed an intervention study aiming at improved psychosocial knowledge in managers (Theorell *et al.* 2001). The managers in an insurance company had mandatory psychosocial education once every second week (half an hour lecture and 90 minutes group discussion) for a whole year. The education programme comprised all relevant aspects of psychosocial working conditions, such as the role of demand, decision latitude, support and effort–reward imbalance. Their employees were examined before, after six months and after one year with regard to psychosocial work conditions and serum cortisol (when they arrived at the office in the morning). Employees in another comparable part of the same organization (whose managers were not subjected to the psychosocial training) were followed at the same intervals (130 subjects in each group). While cortisol remained unchanged in the comparison group, the employees in the intervention group had a substantial and significant decrease in serum cortisol during the follow-up year. There was also a more favourable development of the serum concentration of the liver enzyme gamma glutamyl transferase as well as a more favourable development of serum triglyceride concentration (among women only) in the experimental group, compared to the control group. Both markers are influenced by level of cortisol concentration. Psychosocial questionnaire data from the same groups of employees indicated that the development of decision authority was more favourable in the employees of the intervention group than in the control group while demands and work pace developed in the same way in the two groups. These results indicate that managers could be one target group in psychosocial work site interventions and that improvement of decision authority for employees may be a crucial variable.

Improved manager knowledge may not necessarily be the only possible strategy, however. In a psychosocial intervention programme in Sweden (Orth-Gomér *et al.* 1994) a similar strategy was used which involved all the employees in workplaces. Compared to the control group the intervention group showed improved decision authority and improved lipoprotein patterns.

Bond and Bunce (2001) evaluated the effects of an intervention aiming at improved employee participation in work redesign. In this programme the whole organization was actively involved. The development of mental health, sick leave rate and self-rated performance was significantly better in the intervention group during the year of follow-up than in the comparison group. Further analysis indicated that improved participation among employees in the intervention group was accounting for the favourable development of health in that group.

In summary, while there is some preliminary evidence of beneficial effects on health and well-being produced by theory-based interventions much remains to be done in this field of policy development.

Apart from legal procedures and compensation claims that are increasingly raised in this domain, there are three major incentives of investing into an improved quality of work organization including fair employment contracts (Marmot *et al.* 2005). The first one is responsibility. When asbestos was shown to cause certain types of cancer, preventive steps were taken by occupational health agencies to minimize the risk. A similar case can be made for injury prevention at work. Should we not consider reducing work-related stress as far as scientific evidence tells? Responsibility may not be a convincing argument for some parts of the world's current economy. Yet the European Commission has recently proposed an agenda for Corporate Social Responsibility, and a number of other initiatives support this approach at the global level, such as the ILO's Tripartite Declaration on Multinational Enterprises and Social Policy, and the OECD Guidelines for Multinational Enterprises. In all these initiatives, the protection and promotion of the health of employees is considered an important task of employment policy.

Costs of inactivity define a second incentive. While interest in short-term profit may run against this argument it is nevertheless evident that the costs of an unhealthy work organization create a financial burden to companies and organizations as well as to society at large. A conservative estimate of annual costs of work-related stress in the 15 European Union nations is 20 billion Euro (Dunham 2001). This estimate considers the total sum of direct and indirect health costs of that fraction of the highly prevalent diseases mentioned above that is attributable to work-related stress. This is no more than about 10 per cent of the total variance of these diseases.

Return-on-investment is a third incentive for improving quality of work organization including fair employment contracts. Few studies have been carried out that demonstrate substantial medium-term cost savings of such investments. However, particularly impressive in this regard is a US American study by Jeffery Pfeffer who explored common organizational features of those US companies that were most successful in terms of shareholder value over a number of years (Pfeffer 1998). He came up with the following list of common characteristics:

1 employment security;

2 selective hiring of new personnel;

3 self-managed teams and decentralized decision-making as the basic principles of organizational design;

4 comparatively high compensation contingent on organizational performance;

5 extensive training;

6 reduced status distinctions and barriers across levels; and

7 extensive sharing of financial and performance information throughout the organization.

It is almost certain that Pfeffer was not aware of the models of work stress discussed here, in particular the effort–reward imbalance model and the demand–control model, as his interest was exclusively an economic one. However, it is evident that several of the features of economically successful organizations are similar to those which result as recommendations from the scientific results presented in this chapter.

Therefore, in conclusion, a substantial part of policy implications derived from research on psychosocial stress at work and health concur with these economically driven improvements of work organization including employment contract. Joint efforts are needed from stakeholders, professionals and national/international organizations to further improve the quality of working life and, thus, to reduce social inequalities in health.

References

Ala-Mursula L, Vahtera J, Linna A, Pentti J and Kivinäki M (2005). Employee worktime control moderates the effects of job strain and effort-reward imbalance on sickness absence: the 10-Town Study, *Journal of Epidemiology and Community Health*, **59**, 851–7.

Alderling M, Theorell T, Bergman P, Stoetzer U, de la Torre B and Lundberg I (2005). Saliva cortisol–circadian variation in working men and women in relation to the demand/control model. Manuscript. Dept. of Occupational Health, Karolinska Hospital and National Institute for Psychosocial Factors and Health, Stockholm, Sweden.

Aronsson G, Gustafsson K and Dallner M (2000). Sick but yet at work. An empirical study of sickness presenteeism. *Journal of Epidemiology and Community Health*, **54**, 502–9.

Belkic KL, Landsbergis PA, Schnall PL, Baker D (2004). Is job strain a major source of cardiovascular disease risk? *Scandinavian Journal of Work Environment and Health*, **30**, 85–128.

Benach J, Mutaner C, Benavides FG, Amable M and Jodar P (2002). A new occupational health agenda for a new work environment. *Scandinavian Journal of Work, Environment and Health*, **28**, 191–6.

Blekesaune M and Solem PE (2005). Working conditions and early retirement. A prospective study of retirement behaviour. *Research on Aging*, **7**, 3–30.

Bobak M, Hertzman C, Skodova Z, Marmot M (1998). Association between psychosocial factors at work and non-fatal myocardial infarction in a population based case-control study in Czech men. *Epidemiology*, **9**, 43–47.

Bond FW and Bunce D (2001). Job control mediates change in work organization intervention for stress reduction. *Journal of Occupational Health Psychology*, **6**, 290–302.

Bosma H, Peter R, Siegrist J, Marmot M (1998). Two alternative job stress models and the risk of coronary heart disease. *American Journal of Public Health*, **88**, 68–74.

Breeze E, Fletcher EA, Leon DA, Marmot MG, Clarke RJ and Shipley MJ (2001). Do socioeconomic disadvantages persist into old age? Self-reported morbidity in a 29-year follow-up of the Whitehall Study. *American Journal of Public Health*, **91**, 277–83.

Brisson C, Guimont C, Vézina M *et al.* (2004). Psychosocial work environment and evolution of blood pressure: the contribution of job control and physical work demands. Abstract at the Eighth International Congress of Behavioral Medicine, Mainz, Germany. Available at www.icbm-2004.de

Brunner EJ, Kivimäki M, Siegrist J *et al.* (2004). Is the effect of work stress confounded by socio-economic factors in the Valmet study? *Journal of Epidemiology and Community Health*, **58**, 1019–20.

Cleary AJ (2000). Regulatory disturbance of energy. In: T Theorell (ed.) Everyday biological stress mechanisms. *Advanced Psychosomatic Medicine*, **22**, 17–34.

Collins SM, Karasek RA and Costas K (2004). Job strain and autonomic indices of cardio-vascular disease risk. Eighth International Congress of Behavioral Medicine, Mainz, Germany. Available at www.icbm-2004.de

Cooper CL (ed.) 1998. *Theories of organizational stress*. Oxford University Press, Oxford.

Dragano N, Verde PE and Siegrist J (2005). Organizational downsizing and work stress: testing synergistic health effects in employed men and women. *Journal of Epidemiology and Community Health*, **59**, 694–9.

Dunham J (2001). *Stress in the workplace. Past, present and future*. Whurr, London.

Eaker ED, Sullivan LM, Kelly-Hayes M, D'Agostino RB, Benjamin EJ (2004). Does job strain increase the risk for coronary heart disease or death in men and women? The Framingham Offspring Study. *American Journal of Epidemiology*, **159**, 950–8.

Eurostat (2004). *Work and health in the EU: a statistical portrait*. Luxembourg, Office for Official Publications of the European Communities.

Fujiwara K, Tsukishima E, Kasai S *et al.* (2004). Urinary catecholamines and salivary cortisol on workdays and days off in relation to job strain among female health care providers. *Scandinavian Journal of Work Environment and Health*, **30**, 129–38.

Hallqvist J, Diderichsen F and Theorell T (1998). Is the effect of job strain on myocardial infarction due to interaction between high psychological demands and low decision latitude? Results from the Stockholm Heart Epidemiology Program (SHEEP). *Social Science and Medicine*, **46**, 1405–15.

Hansen AM, Kaergaard A, Andersen JH and Netterstrom B (2003). Associations between repetitive work and endocrinological indicators of stress. *Work and Stress*, 17, 264–76.

Head J, Stansfeld SA, and Siegrist J (2004). The psychosocial work environment and alcohol dependence: a prospective study. *Occupational and Environmental Medicine*, 61, 219–24.

Hemingway H, Shipley M, Stansfeld S and Marmot M (1997). Sickness absence from back pain, psychosocial work characteristics and employment grade among office workers. Whitehall II-Study. *Scandinavian Journal of Work, Environment and Health*, 23, 121–9.

Hertting A and Theorell T (2002). Physiological changes associated with downsizing of personnel and reorganization in the health care sector. *Psychotherapy and Psychosomatics*, 71, 117–22.

Hlatky MA, Lam LC, Lee KL *et al.* (1995). Job strain and the prevalence and outcome of coronary artery disease. *Circulation*, 92, 327–33.

Hoogendoorn WE, Bongers PM, de Vet HC, Ariens GA, van Mechelen W, Bouter LM (2002). High physical work load and low job satisfaction increase the risk of sickness absence due to low back pain: results of a prospective cohort study. *Occupational and Environmental Medicine*, 59, 323–8.

Jeding K, Oxenstierna G, Ferrie J, Westerlund H, Siegrist J and Theorell T (2006). Effort–reward imbalance is associated with increased rates of long-term sickness absence (submitted to *Scandinavian Journal of Public Health*).

Johnson JV and Hall EM (1988). Job strain, workplace social support and cardiovascular disease: a cross-sectional study of a random sample of the Swedish working population. *American Journal of Public Health*, 78, 1336–42.

Joksimovic L, Starke D, Knesebeck O and Siegrist J (2002). Perceived work stress, overcommitment and self-reported musculoskeletal pain a cross-sectional investigation. *International Journal of Behavioral Medicine*, 9, 122–38.

Kaila-Kangas L, Kivimaki M, Riihimaki H, Luukkonen R, Kirjonen J, Leino-Arjas P (2004). Psychosocial factors at work as predictors of hospitalization for back disorders: a 28-year follow-up of industrial employees. *Spine*, 29, 1823–30.

Karasek R (1979). Job demands, job decision latitude, and mental strain: implications for job redesign. *Adminstrative Science Quarterly*, 24, 285–307.

Karasek RA and Theorell T (1990). *Healthy work*. Basic Books, New York.

Kirschbaum C and Hellhammer D (1999). Noise and stress – salivary cortisol as a non-invasive measure of allostatic load. *Noise Health*, 1, 57–66.

Kivimäki M, Hintsanen M, Pulkki L *et al.* (2006). Impact of early life factors on the association between work stress and early atherosclerosis (submitted).

Kivimäki M, Vahtera J, Ferrie JE *et al.* (2001). Organisational downsizing and musculoskeletal problems in employees: a prospective study. *Occupational and Environmental Medicine*, 58, 811–17.

Kompier MA, Aust B, van den Berg AM and Siegrist J (2002). Stress prevention in bus drivers: evaluation of 13 natural experiments. *Journal of Occupational Health Psychology*, 5, 11–31.

Kumari M, Head J, Marmot M (2004). Prospective study of social and other risk factors for incidence of type II diabetes in Whitehall 2 study. *Annals of Internal Medicine*, 164, 1873–80.

Kuper H, Singh-Manoux A, Siegrist J, Marmot M (2002). When reciprocity fails: effort–reward imbalance in relation to coronary heart disease and health functioning within the Whitehall II Study. *Journal of Occupational and Environmental Medicine*, **59**, 777–84.

Landsbergis PA (2003). The changing organization of work and the safety and health of working people: a commentary. *Journal of Occupational and Environmental Medicine*, **11**, 61–71.

Landsbergis PA, Schnall PL, Pickering TG, Warren K and Schwartz JE (2003). Life-course exposure to job strain and ambulatory blood pressure in man. *American Journal of Epidemiology*, **157**, 998–1006.

Larisch M, Joksimovic L, von dem Knesebeck O, Starke D and Siegrist J (2003). Berufliche Gratifikationskrisen und depressive Symptome: eine Querschnittstudie bei Erwerbstätigen im mittleren Erwachsenenalter. *Psychotherapie, Psychosomatik und Medizinische Psychologie*, **53**, 223–8.

Macleod J, Davey Smith G, Heslop P, Metcalfe C, Carroll D and Hart C (2001). Are the effects of psychosocial exposures attributable to confounding? Evidence from a prospective observational study on psychological stress and mortality. *Journal of Epidemiology and Community Health*, **55**, 878–84.

Markovitz JH, Matthews KA, Whooley M, Lewis CE, Greenlund KJ (2004). Increases in job strain are associated with incident hypertension in the CARDIA Study. *Annals of Behavioral Medicine*, **28**, 4–9.

Marmot MG, Bosma H, Hemingway H, Brunner E, Stansfeld S (1997). Contribution of job control and other risk factors to social variations in coronary heart disease. *Lancet*, **350**, 235–40.

Marmot M, Shipley M, Brunner E, Hemingway H (2001). Relative contribution of early life and adult socioeconomic factors to adult morbidity in the Whitehall II study. *Journal of Epidemiology and Community Health*, **55**, 301–7.

Marmot M, Theorell T, Siegrist J (2002). Work and coronary heart disease. In: SA Stansfeld and MG Marmot (eds) *Stress and the heart. Psychosocial pathways to coronary heart disease*, pp. 50–71. BMJ Books, London.

Marmot M, Siegrist J, Theorell T (2005). Health and the psychosocial environment at work. In: M Marmot and RG Wilkinson (eds) *Social determinants of health* 97–130. Oxford University Press, Oxford.

Melchior M, Berkman LF, Kawachi I *et al.* (2006). Lifecourse socioeconomic trajectory predicts non-cardiovascular premature mortality (35–65) among men and women: results from the French GAZEL cohort study. *Journal of Epidemiology and Community Health* (in press)

Mill JS (1848). *Principles of political economy with some of their applications to social philosophy.* (Reprint 1962) Routledge and Kegan Paul, London.

Moreau M, Valente F, Mak R *et al.* (2004). Occupational stress and incidence of sick leave in the Belgian workforce: the Belstress study. *Journal of Epidemiology and Community Health*, **58**, 507–16.

Nettle D (2003). Intelligence and class mobility in the British population. *British Journal of Psychology*, **94**, 551–61.

Niedhammer I, Goldberg M, Leclerc A, Bugel I, David S (1998). Psychosocial factors at work and subsequent depressive symptoms in the Gazel cohort. *Scandinavian Journal of Work Environment and Health*, **24**, 197–205.

Niedhammer I, Siegrist J, Landré MF, Goldberg M, Leclerc A (2000). Étude des qualités psychométriques de la version française du modèle du déséquilibre efforts/ récompenses. *Revue d'Épidémiologie et Santé Publique*, **48**, 419–37.

North F, Symes SL, Feeney A, Shipley M and Marmot M (1996). Psychosocial work environment and sickness absence among British civil servants. The Whitehall II study. *American Journal of Public Health*, **86**, 332–40.

Orth-Gomér K, Eriksson I, Moser V, Theorell T and Fredlund P (1994). Lipid lowering through work stress reduction. *International Journal of Behavioral Medicine*, **1**, 204–14.

Oxenstierna G, Ferrie J, Hyde M, Westerlund H, Theorell T (2005). Dual source support and control at work in relation to health. *Scandinavian Journal of Public Health*, **33**, 455–63.

Perrewe PL and Ganster DC (eds) (2002). *Historical and current perspectives on stress and health*. JAI Elsevier, Amsterdam.

Pfeffer J (1998). *Human equation. Building profit by putting people first*. Harvard Business School Press, Boston, MA.

Pikhart H, Bobak M, Pajak A *et al.* (2004). Psychosocial factors at work and depression in three countries of Central and Eastern Europe. *Social Science and Medicine*, **58**, 1475–82.

Rau R, Georgiades A, Fredrikson M, Lemne C, de Faire (2001). Psychosocial work characteristics and perceived control in relation to cardiovascular rewind at night. *Journal of Occupational Health Psychology*, **6**, 171–81.

Reed DM, La Croix AZ, Karasek RA, Miller D and McLean CA (1989). Occupational strain and the incidence of coronary heart disease. *American Journal of Epidemiology*, **129**, 495–502.

Rosmond R and Bjorntorp P (2000). Occupational status cortisol secretory pattern and visceral obesity in middle-aged men. *Obesity Research*, **8**, 445–50.

Schnall PL, Belkic K, Landsbergis and Baker D (2000). Why the workplace and cardiovascular disease? *Occupational Medicine*, **15**, 1–334.

Siegrist J (1984) Threat to social status and cardiovascular risk. *Psychotherapy and Psychosomatics*, **42**, 90–6.

Siegrist J (1996). Adverse health effects of high-effort/low-reward conditions. *Journal of Occupational Health Psychology*, **1**, 27–41.

Siegrist J, Starke D, Chandola T *et al.* (2004). The measurement of effort–reward imbalance at work: European comparisons. *Social Science and Medicine*, **58**, 1483–99.

Siegrist J, Siegrist K, Weber I (1986). Sociological concepts in the etiology of chronic disease: the case of ischemic heart disease. *Social Science and Medicine*, **22**, 247–53.

Siegrist J, Klein D, Voigt KH (1997). Linking sociological with physiological data: the model of effort–reward imbalance at work. *Acta Physiologica Scandinavia*, **161**, 112–16.

Stansfeld SA and Marmot MG (eds.) (2002). *Stress and the heart*. BMJ Books, London.

Stansfeld SA, Fuhrer R, Shipley MJ, Marmot MG (1999). Work characteristics predict psychiatric disorder: prospective results from the Whitehall II Study. *Occupational and Environmental Medicine*, **56**, 302–7.

Steptoe A, Cropley M, Griffith J, Kirschbaum C (2000). Job strain and anger expression predict early morning elevations in salivary cortisol. *Psychosomatic Medicine*, **62**, 286–92.

Steptoe A, Siegrist J, Kirschbaum C, Marmot M (2004). Effort–reward imbalance, overcommitment, and measures of cortisol and blood pressure over the working day. *Psychosomatic Medicine*, **66**, 323–9.

Steptoe A and Willemsen G (2004). The influence of low job control on ambulatory blood pressure and perceived stress over the working day in men and women from the Whitehall II cohort. *Journal of Hypertension*, **22**, 915–20.

Suadicani P, Hein HO, Gynetelberg F (1993). Are social inequalities as associated with the risk of ischaemic heart disease a result of psychosocial working conditions? *Atherosclerosis*, **101**, 165–75.

Theorell T (2002). Job stress and fibrinogen. Editorial. *European Heart Journal*, **23**, 1799–801.

Theorell T (2004). Democracy at work and its relationship to health. In: PL Perrewé and DC Ganster (eds) *Research in occupational stress and well-being. Emotional and physiological processes and positive intervention strategies*, **3**, pp. 323–57. JAI Elsevier, Amsterdam.

Theorell T, de Faire U, Johnson J, Hall E, Perski A and Stewart W (1991). Job strain and ambulatory blood pressure profiles. *Scandinavian Journal of Work Environment and Health*, **17**, 380–5.

Theorell T, Emdad R, Arnetz B and Weingarten AM (2001). Employee effects of an educational program for managers at an insurance company. *Psychosomatic Medicine*, **63**, 724–33.

Theorell T, Hasselhorn H-M, Vingård E, Andersson B and the MUSIC-Norrtälje Study Group (2000). Interleukin-6 and cortisol in acute musculoskeletal disorders: results from a case-referent study in Sweden. *Stress Medicine*, **16**, 27–35.

Theorell T, Oxenstierna G, Westerlund H, Ferrie J, Hagberg J, Alfredsson L (2003). Downsizing of staff is associated with lowered medically certified sick leave in female employees. *Occupational and Environmental Medicine*, **60**, E9.

Theorell T, Perski A, Åkerstedt T, Sigala F, Ahlberg-Hultén G, Svensson J and Eneroth P (1988). Changes in job strain in relation to changes in physiological state – a longitudinal study. *Scandinavian Journal of Work Environment and Health* **14**, 189–96.

Tsutsumi A, Kawakami N (2004). A review of empirical studies on the model of effort–reward imbalance at work: reducing occupational stress by implementing a new theory. *Social Science and Medicine*, **59**, 2335–59.

Tsutsumi A, Kayaba K, Theorell T and Siegrist J (2001). Association between job stress and depression among Japanese employees threatened by job loss in comparison between two complementary job-stress models. *Scandinavian Journal of Work Environment and Health*, **27**, 147–53.

van Vegchel N, de Jonge J, Bosma H, Schaufeli W (2005). Reviewing the effort-reward imbalance model: drawing up the balance of 45 empirical studies. *Social Science and Medicine*, **60**, 1117–31.

Vahtera J, Kivimäki M, Pentti J et al. (2004). Organisational downsizing, sickness absence. and mortality: 10-town prospective cohort study. *British Medical Journal*, **328**, 555–9.

Vingård E, Alfredsson L, Hagberg M et al. (2000). To what extent do current and past physical and psychosocial occupational factors explain care-seeking for low back pain in a working population? Results from the musculoskeletal intervention centre-Norrtälje study. *Spine*, **25**, 493–500.

Vrijkotte DGM, Doornen LJP van, Geus EJC de (2000). Effect of work stress on ambulatory blood pressure, heart rate, and heart rate variability. *Hypertension*, **35**, 880–6.

Wahlstedt K (2001). Postal work – work organizational changes as tools to improve health. Acta Universitatis Uppsaliensis.

Westerlund H, Ferrie J, Hagberg J, Jeding K, Oxenstierna G, Theorell T (2004a). Workplace expansion, long-term sickness absence, and hospital admission. *Lancet*, **10**, 1193–7.

Westerlund H, Theorell T, Alfredsson L (2004b). Organizational instability and cardiovascular risk factors in white-collar employees: an analysis of correlates of structural instability of workplace organization on risk factors for coronary heart disease in a sample of 3,904 white collar employees in the Stockholm region. *European Journal of Public Health*, **14**, 37–42.

Wigaeus Tornqvist E, Kilbom Å, Alfredsson L *et al.* (2001). The influence on seeking care because of neck and shoulder disorders from work-related exposures. *Epidemiology*, **12**, 537–45.

Chapter 5

Psychobiological processes linking socio-economic position with health

Andrew Steptoe

Introduction

This chapter is concerned with how variations in socio-economic position affect physical disease. There are striking socio-economic disparities in morbidity and mortality from many chronic illnesses, including coronary heart disease, hypertension, diabetes, chronic lung disease, physical disability, some infectious illnesses, and malignancies. As is evident from other chapters in this book, there are several different levels of explanation of socio-economic gradients in disease; economic, life course, social and psychological models all make useful contributions. The topic of this chapter is how socio-economic variations influence biology, and the pathological changes that underlie physical disease. Income, educational attainment, early life disadvantage and other factors do not influence physical pathology directly, but must operate through more proximal mechanisms. In order to understand the magnitude of socio-economic determinants and how their effects might be ameliorated, we need to know what pathways translate the life experience of different social groups into varying levels of pathology. The main emphasis in this chapter will be on coronary heart disease and related cardiovascular disorders, though other diseases are also discussed.

The chapter begins by describing the pathways that theoretically link socio-economic position with physical disease, and by explaining the potential significance of psychobiological responses. The findings concerning psychobiological processes are organized round the primary methodologies that have been used to explore these pathways, namely animal studies, human laboratory mental stress testing, and naturalistic studies of biological function in everyday life. It will become apparent that there has been rapid development in this field over recent years, and that although there are still many uncertainties, we are moving into an era in which conclusions about the significance of psychobiological processes can be made with greater confidence.

Pathways to disease

There are a number of pathways through which variations in socio-economic position might theoretically lead to differences in the likelihood that an individual acquires a physical illness. One possibility is that there are socio-economic variations in exposure to infectious agents or chemical hazards. Many diseases of poverty arise from infections or toxic factors related to poor water supplies, unhygienic living conditions and industrial pollution. Such exposure might be important not only for explaining the health impact of poverty, but also for variations across the social gradient. For example, certain groups such as people working in the textile industry are exposed to carbon disulphide which stimulates increased low-density lipoprotein (LDL)-cholesterol and raised blood pressure (Egeland *et al.* 1992). Lifetime infection with micro-organisms may elicit chronic low level inflammation that contributes to the progression of atherosclerosis (Kiechl *et al.* 2001). Acute infection may also stimulate transient increases in vascular events such as myocardial infarction or stroke (Smeeth *et al.* 2004). But although infectious processes may plausibly be related to socio-economic position, no evidence directly linking infection with the gradient in cardiovascular or other chronic diseases has yet been published.

A stronger case can be made for the role of health behaviours such as smoking, physical activity, food choice and alcohol intake in mediating socio-economic gradients. Many aspects of healthy lifestyle correlate with socio-economic position, and behavioural pathways are certainly responsible for some of the variation in the incidence of physical diseases (Wardle *et al.* 1999). The best example is smoking and lung cancer. Since smoking is a primary determinant of lung cancer, in countries in which there is a social gradient in smoking, it is clearly the main factor underlying socio-economic variations in lung cancer incidence. But generalizations about the role of health behaviours in socio-economic health gradients in other diseases are difficult to make. The importance of health behaviours and lifestyle factors varies greatly between medical conditions. While it is true that people in higher socio-economic positions are more prudent in many health behaviours, this is not always the case. For example, the socio-economic gradient in dietary fat consumption is weak and inconsistent (Dowler 2001), greater alcohol consumption in more affluent groups has been described in some studies (Hulshof *et al.* 2003), and socio-economic gradients in smoking and fruit and vegetable consumption vary across countries (Cavelaars *et al.* 1997). Some attempts have been made to quantify the extent to which health behaviours contribute to socio-economic gradients in mortality in particular cohorts, and estimates of between 30 and 60 per cent have emerged (Lantz *et al.* 2001, Schrijvers *et al.* 1999, Van Lenthe *et al.* 2002). These findings suggest that behavioural pathways play a major role in mediating the socio-economic gradient of some pathologies, but that they are only part of the story.

Psychobiological processes

Psychobiological processes are the pathways through which psychosocial factors stimulate biological systems via central nervous system activation of autonomic, neuroendocrine, immune and inflammatory responses (Steptoe and Ayers 2004). Structures in the limbic system (notably the amygdala) operate in conjunction with the prefrontal cortex to control lower brain processes regulating peripheral physiological activity. The biological responses that are particularly relevant to disease are organized through two neurobiological pathways: the hypothalamic–pituitary–adrenocortical (HPA) axis leading to the release of hormones such as cortisol, and the sympathoadrenal axis, involving stimulation of the sympathetic branch of the autonomic nervous system in conjunction with hormones such as adrenaline (epinephrine) and noradrenaline (norepinephrine). These pathways have a range of effects on peripheral tissues. For example, cortisol stimulates the production of glucose in the liver, helps release free fatty acids from fat stores, and is involved in the regulation of water balance and the control of the immune system. Sympathetic nervous system activation leads to increases in blood pressure and heart rate, stimulation of blood clotting factors, upregulation of immune function, and release of stored free fatty acids. When these systems are exposed to repeated or chronic stimulation, dysregulation that can have adverse effects on health may ensue.

There is extensive evidence from studies of animals conducted over the past 40 years that prolonged or intensive stimulation of these psychobiological pathways can increase pathology both directly, and by impairing host resistance, thereby allowing infectious agents and other pathogens to proliferate (Henry and Stephens 1977, Weiner 1992). The conditions studied have included both unpleasant laboratory stressors and naturalistic situations such as being hunted (Bateson and Bradshaw 1997). Some of the most compelling work has involved social stressors rather than painful or frightening conditions. For example, Henry and co-workers (Henry *et al.* 1975) showed that conflict induced by raising mice first in isolation and then introducing them into structured social environments calculated to encourage interaction, resulted in acute elevations of blood pressure that subsequently became sustained and irreversible with prolonged exposure. Kaplan and colleagues

(1983) have conducted a series of studies of social stress and coronary athero-sclerosis in cynomolgus macaques. Stress induced by periodic disruption of social hierarchies resulted in accelerated coronary atherosclerosis, vascular endothelial dysfunction, increased susceptibility to infection, and deposition of abdominal fat, albeit with important gender differences (Cohen *et al.* 1997, Jayo *et al.* 1993, Williams *et al.* 1993). It is important to note in these studies that individual animals vary markedly in their susceptibility, and that this variation is correlated with autonomic reactivity to emotional stress (Manuck *et al.* 1983). In humans as well, individual differences in psychobiological responsivity to adverse experiences need to be taken into account.

Animal studies have also shown that psychobiological responses are associ-ated with dominance hierarchies. Working with wild olive baboons, Sapolsky (1990) established that basal cortisol levels are higher in subordinate animals, and in the female cynomolgus macaques, social subordination also leads to stimulation of the HPA axis and is associated with increased coronary athero-sclerosis (Shively and Clarkson 1994). However, the analogy with social gradi-ents in humans can be overstated. As Kaplan and Manuck (1999) have pointed out, there is nothing inherently pathogenic in either subordinate or dominant social status in animals. In male cynomolgus monkeys, coronary atherosclero-sis is greater in dominant than subordinate animals under unstable social con-ditions, while the pattern is reversed in females. In baboons, the pattern of higher cortisol in subordinates is only present under stable conditions, and not when social hierarchies are disrupted. A broad overview of social rank dif-ferences in cortisol levels in many different primate species has highlighted the variability of effects (Abbott *et al.* 2003). For example, cortisol levels are lower in subordinates than dominants in cotton top tamarins, at a similar level in male rhesus monkeys, but are higher in dominant than subordinate female cynomolgus and male squirrel monkeys. It appears that subordinates have higher relative cortisol levels in species in which dominance hierarchies are maintained by overt aggression, and where there is little social support for subordinates. These subtleties highlight the need for precision in defining the factors sustaining social hierarchies.

Psychobiological responses, allostasis and individual differences

If psychobiological pathways do mediate, at least in part, socio-economic dis-parities in physical health, what sort of responses are involved? It is significant that the psychosocial factors that are thought to increase risk of chronic pathologies such as the progression of coronary atherosclerosis, hypertension and type 2 diabetes, are not acute traumatic stressors or major life events.

Rather, they are conditions that can endure for many years such as chronic work stress, social isolation, family conflict and depressed mood. Such factors are not likely to produce major disturbances of psychobiological response, but rather low-level disruption and dysregulation. This is one reason why the concepts of allostasis and allostatic load have been attractive to researchers of socio-economic factors and health. Allostasis was a term introduced by Sterling and Eyer (1988) to describe how the cardiovascular system adjusts to different behavioural states, and means maintaining stability and home-ostasis through change. It has been elaborated primarily by McEwen (1998), who developed the notion of allostatic load. This refers to the wear and tear imposed on biological regulatory systems as they are forced to adapt repeatedly to life's demands. Over time, chronic allostatic load can lead to reduced adaptability, and the failure of systems to remain within optimal operating ranges. McEwen has argued that allostatic load can have several different effects on bodily systems, including failure to habituate to repeated stimulation, failure of post-stress recovery, and failure to mount an adequate biological response in the face of challenge at all. Chronic allostatic load has been implicated in a number of health-related settings including mood disorders (McEwen 2003) and the maintenance of cognitive and physiological functioning in old age (Seeman *et al.* 2001), as well as in socio-economic inequalities (McEwen and Seeman 1999).

There are two elements of the allostatic load approach that are particularly relevant for studies of psychobiology and socio-economic position. The first is the emphasis on small changes in biological response. Differences in blood pressure of a few millimetres, or in interleukin (IL) 6 of one or two pg/L, may be significant if they are sustained over months and years. Second, the allostatic model focuses attention on recovery effects, and on the rate at which biological responses return to reference levels after challenge. As will become clear, this aspect is especially important in comparisons of socio-economic groups.

The individual differences evident in animal studies are very striking in humans as well. If several people are exposed to the same psychological challenge, such as carrying out a problem-solving task under time pressure, they will show a wide range of cardiovascular, neuroendocrine and inflammatory responses. These differences may be due to gain (amplification) at several levels of the psychobiological response system, including the prefrontal/limbic level, the hypothalamic/brainstem level, the sensitivity of peripheral organs and tissues, and the sensitivity of physiological feedback systems (Lovallo 2004). Individual differences are determined by a combination of genetic factors, early life experiences, background stress levels, coping and appraisal processes (Steptoe and Ayers 2004). The important question is whether socio-economic position also influences psychobiological processes.

Mental stress testing studies

One important method that has been used to discover whether low socio-economic position is associated with psychobiological dysregulation is laboratory mental stress testing. This involves the measurement of biological responses while people are exposed to demanding situations such as problem-solving tasks, emotionally stressful interviews, or simulated public speaking. The methodological strengths of this approach have been rehearsed extensively (Steptoe and Vögele 1991). First, all individuals are exposed to exactly the same challenge. Consequently, variations in the magnitude or patterning of biological changes are due to variations in response and not to differences in stimulation. This situation rarely pertains in everyday life, where people's exposures to challenge vary markedly. Second, measurement of complex physiological and biological parameters can be carried out under highly controlled conditions. When biological measurements are carried out in everyday life or during epidemiological surveys, it is seldom feasible to obtain more than rather simple measures. Third, potential confounding factors can be monitored or eliminated, so that conclusions about differences in responsivity can be made with greater confidence.

Mental stress testing typically involves administration of relatively brief challenges lasting 5–20 minutes. There are two major components to the psychobiological response: the size of the response, and the speed of post-task recovery. One individual or group might produce larger blood pressure or plasma fibrinogen increases than another in response to tasks, or could produce the same size of response but vary in the rate at which the biological measure returns to baseline levels. Both these factors are thought to be significant for disease pathology. For example, variations in acute blood pressure reactions have been shown to predict future hypertension and the progression of subclinical atherosclerosis (Treiber *et al.* 2003). Jennings *et al.* (2004) studied 756 men from the Kuopio Ischemic Heart Disease Study, measuring blood pressure and heart rate responses to a battery of challenging tasks including colour-word interference and mirror tracing. Carotid intima-media thickness (IMT) was assessed as a marker of atherosclerosis at the time of stress testing and again seven years later. The magnitude of systolic blood pressure reactions to mental stress tests was positively associated with later carotid IMT, and to progression of subclinical atherosclerosis between testing sessions, even after controlling for resting blood pressure, initial IMT levels, lipid levels, age and education. Similarly, slow rates of post-stress recovery have been associated with increased cardiovascular disease risk (Laukkanen *et al.* 2004, Schuler and O'Brien 1997).

Laboratory mental stress testing has been used to elucidate the role of many psychosocial factors in physical disease risk, including social support and social isolation (Uchino *et al.* 1996), hostility and type A behaviour (Miller *et al.* 1996), chronic life stress (Gump and Matthews 1999), and job strain and job control (Siegrist *et al.* 1997, Steptoe *et al.* 1993). In each of these cases, there is some evidence that higher levels of the psychosocial risk factor are associated with greater biological stress reactivity or slower post-stress recovery. We can therefore hypothesize that lower socio-economic position might also be associated with greater reactivity or impaired recovery.

A small number of studies have been carried out on this topic in the past, with somewhat mixed results. For example, Owens *et al.* (1993) studied 49 men and women aged 40–55 years, and found that systolic and diastolic blood pressure and heart rate reactions to a simulated public speaking task were greater in people of lower educational attainment. An analysis of results from the Kuopio study showed that high systolic blood pressure reactivity (defined as the change occurring in anticipation on an exercise test) was more common in less educated men (Lynch *et al.* 1998). By contrast, two studies from the UK showed the reverse pattern. Carroll *et al.* (1997) analysed data from 1091 male civil servants from the Whitehall II cohort who performed a problem-solving task in the presence of aversive noise. Systolic pressure reactivity was greater in higher than lower-status participants, as defined by grade of employment. In a second study, Carroll and colleagues (2000) found that diastolic pressure and heart rate reactions were greater in non-manual than manual workers in a cohort of 1657 men and women aged 23–63. Cardiovascular reactivity appears to be related to lower socio-economic position more consistently in studies of adolescents, although with some important ethnic differences (Barnes *et al.* 2000, Gump *et al.* 1999, Wilson *et al.* 2000).

However, these studies of psychobiological responsivity and socio-economic position are limited by three factors. First, the focus has been exclusively on stress reactivity and not on rate of recovery. If low socio-economic position induces a state of chronic allostatic load, one might anticipate important differences in the post-stress recovery period. The second difficulty relates to the type of tasks administered during mental stress testing. It is essential that tasks are appraised similarly by people across the social gradient. A cardinal principle of physiological mental stress testing is that reactions are associated with engagement and involvement with the challenge (Singer 1974). If one group feels more stressed or challenged by tasks than another, then their responses will be altered. Many of the tasks used in mental stress testing have been adaptations of intelligence tests, so people of different intellectual capacity may not have been engaged to the same extent (Carroll *et al.* 1997, 2000, Rose *et al.* 2004). In the same way, public speaking is much more familiar to people in higher socio-economic positions who may speak to small groups or larger audiences as part of their regular work, so simulated public speaking tasks are inappropriate. In studying socio-economic differences, it is important to administer challenges that are appraised similarly across the gradient, and to measure these appraisals directly in order to ensure that there are no systematic differences. These factors may confound the results of social status group comparisons. For example, Kapuku *et al.* (2002) found in a study of young black men that low socio-economic status was associated with low diastolic blood pressure stress reactivity, but it also emerged that these lower-status men were less involved and engaged in the tasks. The third limitation is that the focus has been almost exclusively on blood pressure and heart rate, with very little work on other measures (Evans *et al.* 2000, Hellhammer *et al.* 1997). The interest of our research group is in the development of coronary artery disease, so we thought it important to include measures of biological processes directly involved in the atherosclerotic process.

Coronary atherosclerosis is a chronic inflammatory condition, rather than a passive lipid storage disease (Lusis 2000, Ross 1999). The inflammation begins in the endothelial lining of vessel walls, and leads to the adhesion of white blood cells (monocytes, lymphocytes, and platelets) to the wall, and migration into the subendothelial intimal layer. The endothelium becomes more permeable to lipoproteins such as LDL-cholesterol that accumulate in the subendothelial matrix, where monocytes differentiate into macrophages and scavenge oxidized LDL to form foam cells. Subsequently, there is a migration and proliferation of smooth muscle cells from outer layers of blood vessel walls into the intimal layer, and the production of extracellular fibrous matrix tissue. These processes are regulated by adhesion molecules and inflammatory cytokines such as IL-6 and tumor necrosis factor (TNF) α, while inflammatory proteins such as C-reactive protein are also involved. At later stages of the disease process, plaques form on the internal vessel wall and undergo repeated disruption through rupture or erosion (Davies 1996). Blood clotting or haemostatic factors such as Von Willebrand factor, factor VIII, plasma viscosity and fibrin D-dimer are therefore also involved.

Several of these inflammatory processes are sensitive to acute mental stress and are associated with psychosocial risk factors. We have therefore sought to include them in psychobiological studies of socio-economic position.

Whitehall psychobiological studies

The principal psychobiological studies of socio-economic position that we have carried out have involved London-based civil servants. The main study included 238 middle-aged men and women who were sampled by grade of employment from the Whitehall II epidemiological cohort. This cohort was originally recruited in 1985–88 to investigate demographic, psychosocial and biological risk factors for coronary heart disease (Marmot *et al.* 1991). The advantage of including Whitehall cohort members is that grade of employment in the British civil service is known to be related to heart disease. Thus by systematically sampling from higher, intermediate and lower grades, we can identify groups varying on socio-economic characteristics known to be relevant to physical health. Grade of employment is closely related to other markers of socio-economic position such as income, educational attainment, and subjective social status (Singh-Manoux *et al.* 2003). We have also carried out studies involving civil servants who are not members of the Whitehall II cohort, but work in equivalent grades.

We piloted a number of behavioural tasks to select tests that were performed to a similar standard across grades of employment, and which were appraised as similarly stressful, involving, difficult and uncontrollable by people of higher and lower social status. This resulted in the choice of two moderate but not severely stressful brief tasks, a computerized colour/word interference task, and mirror tracing. Subjective appraisals and objective performance of these tasks do not vary with grade of employment (Steptoe *et al.* 2002). Our strategy has been to carry out cardiovascular monitoring continuously during pre-task baselines, the tasks themselves, and then during the post-task recovery period for up to two hours. Blood samples are drawn periodically to assess immediate responses to the stressors, and then the recovery effects.

The results of these experiments are summarized in Table 5.1, where three different types of socio-economic effect are described. The first pattern is of socio-economic difference in stress reactivity, and we have observed this in rather few variables. Systolic and diastolic blood pressure reactivity were greater in lower than higher grade of employment groups, but this pattern was present only in women and not men (Steptoe *et al.* 2002). The gender difference is interesting, since the previous studies that have failed to show heightened blood pressure reactivity in lower socio-economic groups have mainly been carried out with men (Carroll *et al.* 1997, Kapuku *et al.* 2002). More interestingly, a greater increase in plasma IL-6 has been recorded from lower occupational grade participants (Brydon *et al.* 2004). Cytokines such as IL-6 respond slowly to behavioural challenge, so this difference does not emerge until two hours post-stress. Interleukin-6 is expressed by many tissues including muscle and fat depots, and it is possible that the stress-induced

Table 5.1 Mental stress testing and socio-economic position

Larger stress reactions in lower socio-economic status participants

♦ Interleukin-6

♦ Systolic and diastolic blood pressure (women only)

Impaired post-stress recovery in lower socio-economic status participants

♦ Systolic and diastolic blood pressure

♦ Heart rate

♦ Heart rate variability

♦ Factor VIII

♦ Plasma viscosity

♦ Blood viscosity

Higher stress levels in lower socio-economic status participants, but no difference in reactivity or recovery

♦ Plasma fibrinogen

♦ Von Willebrand factor

♦ Platelet activation

♦ Tumour necrosis factor α

♦ Interleukin-1 receptor antagonist

♦ Natural killer cell counts

♦ Haematocrit

increase is due to release of the cytokine into the circulation. However, we have recently found that stress stimulates IL-1β gene expression in peripheral mononuclear blood cells, and that this effect is in turn correlated with the increase in plasma IL-6 (Brydon *et al.* 2005). We therefore have reason to believe that lower socio-economic position may stimulate higher levels of inflammatory cytokine gene expression, and not merely changes in concentration between bodily compartments.

A more common pattern of socio-economic difference is found in the rate of post-stress recovery. As shown in Table 5.1, there are socio-economic differences in recovery of systolic and diastolic blood pressure, heart rate and heart rate variability, factor VIII (part of the clotting cascade), plasma viscosity and blood viscosity (Brydon *et al.* 2004, Steptoe *et al.* 2002, 2003c). In each case, lower employment grade participants showed less effective post-stress recovery and return to reference levels. These effects were quite substantial. For example, the odds of incomplete recovery 45 minutes after stress in lower compared with higher grade participants were 2.60 (95 per cent C.I. 1.20 to 5.65) for systolic and 3.85 (1.48 to 10.0) for diastolic blood pressure, adjusted for gender, age, baseline values and the magnitude of reactions to tasks. Differences were present not only in cardiovascular measures, but also in factors related to haemostatis and thrombus formation. Since high viscosity is a risk factor for future coronary heart disease (Danesh *et al.* 2000), these findings suggest that levels may be elevated for longer periods in lower social status groups in response to everyday challenges, thereby increasing disease risk.

The third pattern of response observed in our acute stress studies is higher levels of the biological measure during stress in the lower status groups, but no differences in reactivity or recovery. This pattern is illustrated in Figure 5.1 in a study of platelet activation indexed by leukocyte-platelet aggregates (Steptoe *et al.* 2003d). The proportion of leukocyte-platelet aggregates assessed using flow cytometry has been recommended as a more precise measure of platelet activation than other markers, since it involves minimal manipulation of cells, so the danger of artefactual activation is reduced (Michelson *et al.* 2001). As can be seen in Figure 5.1, platelet activation was elevated in the lower social status group not only during stress, but also during baseline and recovery periods. Higher levels of function were therefore observed throughout the session in lower status participants, so that even though both groups responded to tasks with increased activation, the increase did not vary with socio-economic position. Similar patterns were recorded in several other haemostatic, inflammatory and immune markers (Owen *et al.* 2003, Steptoe *et al.* 2003a, 2003c).

One important omission from Table 5.1 is neuroendocrine function, and in particular cortisol. The reason is that cortisol has not proved to be very responsive to the mental stress tests we have used, so individual differences in the magnitude of reactions are small (Kunz-Ebrecht *et al.* 2003). It is probable that more intense forms of acute challenge involving interpersonal threat are

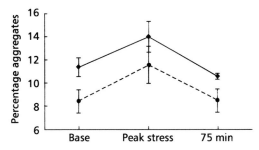

Figure 5.1 Mean percentage of monocyte-platelet aggregates from baseline, peak stress and 75 min post-stress blood samples, in men from higher social status (dashed line) and lower social status (solid line) groups. Values are adjusted for age, and error bars are standard errors of the mean (SEM). From Steptoe *et al.* (2003d).

required to produce marked cortisol reactions (Dickerson and Kemeny 2004). Kristenson *et al.* (2001) reported that plasma cortisol responses to acute stress were smaller in lower than higher social status men in Vilnius (Lithuania) and Linköping (Sweden), a pattern that is the reverse of what we have observed for other variables. The stress tests used in this study were a combination of anger recall, mental arithmetic and pain stimulation procedures, and are rather different from many mental stress procedures carried out in this field.

In summary, these laboratory findings suggest that low socio-economic position is associated with disturbances of psychobiological regulation, and with heightened levels of biological markers of disease risk. Dysfunction is most apparent during post-stress recovery periods, as would be predicted by the allostatic load model. However, current work has a number of limitations. First, measures are taken only of acute responses to short-term challenge, and these effects may be different from those observed under conditions of chronic strain. Second, the challenges imposed are arbitrary, and not clearly relevant to socio-economic position; people do not go about their everyday lives carrying out colour-word interference tasks. I have argued elsewhere it is important to develop challenges that are directly relevant to the psychosocial factor under consideration (Steptoe 1985). Third, results are cross-sectional, and have been obtained during a single laboratory session. They may therefore not be significant for the development of physical pathology and the mediation of socio-economic health variations.

One way of addressing these issues is to test the relationship of acute response patterns to the progression of chronic risk in a longitudinal fashion. As noted earlier, there is evidence that blood pressure stress reactivity predicts future risk of hypertension (Treiber *et al.* 2003). In a three-year follow up of our Whitehall psychobiology study, we have found that impaired post-stress blood pressure recovery predicted increases in clinical blood pressure independently of covariates (Steptoe and Marmot 2005a).

Less is known about the significance of stress responsivity or recovery in other biological variables. Steptoe and Brydon (2005) tested the signific-ance of acute stress-induced increases in lipids on later fasting lipid levels. The magnitude of stress reactivity in total, LDL-cholesterol, and total/HDL-cholesterol ratio predicted three year fasting levels of these lipids, independently of baseline values, age, gender, change in body mass index, smoking and alcohol consumption. We also have some evidence for the significance of acute inflammatory stress responses. Brydon and Steptoe (2005) analysed changes in ambulatory blood pressure over a three year period in 153 men and women. The first day of ambulatory blood pressure monitoring took place around the same time as laboratory mental stress testing. We found that ambulatory systolic blood pressure on three year follow-up was independently predicted by the magnitude of plasma fibrinogen and IL-6 stress responses. These effects are illustrated in Figure 5.2, where ambulatory systolic pressure averaged over the day and evening is plotted for individuals in the lowest, medium, and highest tertiles of fibrinogen and IL-6 stress response. The differences in follow-up blood pressure were independent of baseline ambulatory blood pressure (itself a strong predictor of three year levels), and also of acute blood pressure stress responsivity, resting blood pressure baseline levels, baseline fibrinogen and IL-6, age, gender, smoking and body mass index. The findings indicate that inflammatory responses to acute mental stress may be significant for future cardiovascular health.

What we have not been able to do thus far is to link variations in acute biological stress reactivity or recovery with socio-economic differences in disease risk longitudinally. The reason is that sample sizes have been too small

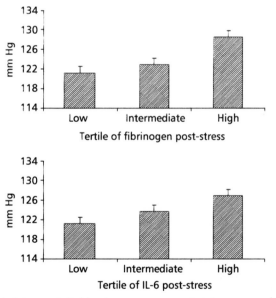

Figure 5.2 Ambulatory systolic blood pressure assessed at three years after mental stress testing. The upper panel shows levels of systolic pressure in relation to fibrinogen stress responses, with the sample divided into low, intermediate and high fibrinogen stress reactors. Values are adjusted for baseline ambulatory systolic pressure, systolic pressure stress responsivity, gender, age, body weight, smoking, and baseline fibrinogen. The lower panel shows follow-up ambulatory systolic pressure in relation to IL-6 stress responses, adjusted for the baseline IL-6 and the other factors listed above. Error bars are SEM. From Brydon and Steptoe (2005).

to show such effects with any confidence. It is hoped that future studies will be of sufficient magnitude to test these effects directly.

Monitoring of biological markers in everyday life

Naturalistic studies of physiological activity in everyday life provide an opportunity to assess the ways in which people's social and emotional experience directly influence their biology. Instead of recording responses to arbitrary stimuli in the restricted environment of the laboratory or clinic, naturalistic monitoring allows people to carry out their normal round of activities, work and social interaction. This area of research has progressed greatly over recent years because of two advances. The first was the development of lightweight ambulatory blood pressure monitors and Holter monitors for heart rate. These devices permit cardiovascular activity to be recorded repeatedly over both day and night with comparatively little interference. The second was the adaptation of biochemical analyses to saliva that have enabled neuroendocrine function to be assessed repeatedly in everyday life. Before this technology was available, it was necessary to collect urine or take blood samples in order to measure cortisol and hormones such as testosterone and dehydroepiandrosterone (DHEA). Studies of the diurnal rhythm of cortisol output used to require heroic processes such as hourly blood draws from indwelling cannulae over 24 hours (Van Cauter *et al.* 2000). These hormones can now be measured from saliva samples taken by participants themselves at designated times, and the substances remain relatively stable for several days (Kirschbaum and Hellhammer 2000).

Unfortunately, naturalistic methods have a number of limitations. The first is that the range of biological markers that can be assessed is small compared with that available in the laboratory, so detailed investigation of factors related to physical pathology is restricted. Most studies to date have involved measures of blood pressure, heart rate and heart rate variability, and salivary cortisol, although new methods for assessing detailed haemodynamics have also been developed. Second, analysing the relationship of ambulatory data with psychosocial factors is complicated, since several influences have to be taken into account. Physical activity, smoking, time of day, eating and drinking caffeinated beverages all affect physiological function, and need to be incorporated into statistical models. A third more subtle problem is that people may adjust their activities during a period of naturalistic monitoring, so that it is no longer typical for them. In a study of school teachers, we measured physical activity using accelerometers on one normal day, and a second day on which ambulatory blood pressure monitoring was carried out (Costa *et al.* 1999).

Physical activity levels were significantly lower on the blood pressure monitoring day, and participants were also more limited in what they did; they were less likely, for example, to be out in the evening, and tended to stay quietly at home.

Hypothetical relationships

The application of naturalistic monitoring to our understanding of the biology of socio-economic position is still at an early stage of scientific development. However, it is worth considering the different types of relationship that might hypothetically link socio-economic position with biological function in everyday life. There are at least three possibilities:

1 *Differences in level of function.* It is conceivable that socio-economic groups vary in their levels of physiological function in everyday life in ways that are related to disease risk. Ambulatory blood pressure level predicts future cardiovascular disease independently of office or clinic levels (Verdecchia 2000), and low heart rate variability is an independent predictor of all cause mortality (Dekker *et al.* 2000). If these patterns are more prominent in lower social status groups, it might explain part of the social gradient in disease risk.

2 *Differences in rhythm.* It is possible that lower socio-economic position might disrupt the normal diurnal rhythms of physiological function. For example, certain forms of chronic stress are associated with a flattening of the usual cortisol decline over the day (Adam and Gunnar 2001). The cortisol response to waking (the increase that takes place over the first 30–60 minutes of the day) can be associated with chronic strain even when the rest of the day is unaffected (Kunz-Ebrecht *et al.* 2004, Steptoe *et al.* 2000). Such effects may be present even when average levels are unchanged, and may reflect persistent challenges to adaptive mechanisms or chronic allostatic load.

3 *Differences in responses to events.* Psychosocial studies involving naturalistic monitoring depend on exposure to adversity. In contrast to the situation in laboratory testing when all participants are exposed to the same stimuli, people have a range of experiences during their everyday lives. Lower socio-economic position is characterized by greater exposure to chronic life stressors in the domains of work, family and emotional life, and in financial and economic areas (Mirowsky and Ross 2003, Turner *et al.* 1995). It is possible, therefore, that social inequalities stimulate differences in the frequency and magnitude of responses to everyday hassles. It is

known, for instance, that blood pressure is slightly elevated during periods of low controllability and social conflict (Kamarck *et al.* 1998), while stressful daily events lead to heightened cortisol secretion (van Eck *et al.* 1996).

These different hypothetical relationships between socio-economic position and physiology in everyday life need to be studied with different analytic strategies; for example, the identification of transient responses to events will not be possible if records are averaged over lengthy periods of time. Clear conceptual models are therefore needed. Additionally, it should be borne in mind that effects are likely to be small. Even in the area of work stress and ambulatory blood pressure where robust effects have been observed for many years, differences between high and low job strain group amount to only a few millimetres mercury pressure (Schnall *et al.* 1994). It is important to recognize that the effects observed during naturalistic monitoring are not usually direct manifestations of pathology, but indications of physiological dysregulation. Their importance lies in the fact that they are typical for that individual, so may be repeated on a regular basis for months or even years. We have previously drawn the analogy with cigarette smoking (Steptoe and Marmot 2005b). A single cigarette has an acute effect on biological function that soon dissipates with no lasting consequences. But a cigarette every thirty minutes, every day, every month, every year for decades has a profound effect on health. The same may apply to the responses observed in psychobiological studies.

Blood pressure and heart rate

There have been relatively few direct comparisons of socio-economic groups using ambulatory blood pressure or heart rate assessments, and results have been rather inconsistent. An investigation of mild hypertensives found that blood pressure levels over the working day and evening were greater in higher status participants (Blumenthal *et al.* 1995), while in another study blood pressure levels were slightly greater in lower status men (Light *et al.* 1995). Matthews *et al.* (2000) compared ambulatory blood pressure and heart rate measures in 50 high and 50 lower-status university employees. There were no differences in systolic or diastolic pressure over working or non-working days, but heart rates were higher in those lower-status participants who reported negative moods over the day. In the Whitehall psychobiology study, we found that systolic blood pressure was 5–6 mmHg greater in the lower grade of employment group after adjusting for age, gender, smoking, alcohol intake, physical activity and body weight (Steptoe *et al.* 2003b). But this difference was only apparent in the morning, and not over the remainder of the day.

However, ambulatory blood pressure is influenced by chronic stress. Research on job strain has already been mentioned, but relationships between elevated blood pressure and marital conflict and care-giver strain have also been recorded (Baker *et al.* 1999, King *et al.* 1994). Our group has recently found that marital strain indexed with the marital/ partner role quality scales was associated with elevated diastolic pressure over the day in a working sample (Barnett *et al.* 2005). There is some evidence that exposure to these sources of chronic stress might lead to differential cardiovascular responses across the social gradient. Landsbergis *et al.* (2003) asked whether the impact of job strain on blood pressure was related to socio-economic position in a work site project in New York City. They found that the effect of job strain was large in lower socio-economic status men defined by education or occupation, and was minimal in higher status men.

An analysis from the Whitehall psychobiology study has also shown different ambulatory blood pressure responses to work-related factors in higher and lower status participants. In collaboration with Siegrist, we assessed the impact of overcommitment, the cognitive and motivational pattern of coping with work demands that is characterized by work-related preoccupation and inability to switch off (Steptoe *et al.* 2004b). We found that overcommitment had a particularly deleterious impact on the systolic blood pressure of lower-status men as defined by grade of employment. The results summarized in Figure 5.3 show that as the working day progresses, systolic pressure increased in overcommitted men, but declined slightly in the non-overcommitted group. The differences were significant in the afternoon and evening periods after controlling for age, smoking, body mass, physical activity, and job control. Interestingly, the other element of Siegrist's model of work stress,

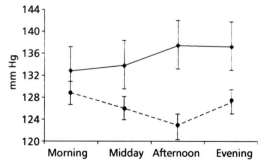

Figure 5.3 Systolic blood pressure recorded over the working day in men working in lower status jobs and reporting high (solid line) and low (dotted line) levels of overcommitment. The day is divided into four time periods. Error bars are SEM. From Steptoe *et al.* (2004b).

effort–reward imbalance, has been related to elevated heart rate and reduced parasympathetic or vagal tone in a sample of male non-manual workers (Vrijkotte *et al.* 2000).

Cortisol profiles

Cortisol plays a central role in stress processes, and HPA dysregulation is one of the cardinal features of the allostatic load model. However, studies of cortisol profiles in everyday life in relation to socio-economic position have shown mixed results to date. There are several reasons for this. First, since cortisol varies widely across the day, the timing of comparisons is critical. Some studies have used single measures, while others have assessed the patterns of change over particular parts of the day described earlier. Second, it is vital to take into account the influence of other factors known to affect cortisol levels; for instance, the concentration of cortisol measured from a single sample at 9.00 a.m. may be different for someone who wakes at 6.30 a.m. or at 8.00 a.m. Third, disturbances of HPA axis function may be present even in the absence of consistent differences in cortisol level. Cortisol values in plasma, saliva and urine depend not only on secretion rates, but also on tissue clearance and effective signalling and receptor sensitivity (Raison and Miller 2003). This is illustrated by studies of HPA axis function in obesity, where greater abdominal adiposity is characterized by altered enzyme function in the liver and fat depots, and by altered central nervous system regulation, without consistent differences in plasma cortisol being present through the day (Seckl *et al.* 2004). These factors may account for the inconsistent associations between socio-economic position and cortisol sampled in everyday life that have been reported to date (Brandtstadter *et al.* 1991, Lupien *et al.* 2000, Rosmond and Bjorntorp 2000, Steptoe *et al.* 2003b).

Recent research suggests that the cortisol response to waking may be a particularly sensitive marker of chronic strain and HPA dysregulation. Cortisol responses to waking are greater on work days compared with weekends, in people experiencing chronic work stress, and in those reporting depression and loneliness (Pruessner *et al.* 1997, 2003, Schlotz *et al.* 2004, Steptoe *et al.* 2004a). By contrast, chronic fatigue and physical illness appear to be associated with a diminished cortisol response to waking (Kudielka and Kirschbaum 2003, Roberts *et al.* 2004). In analyses of our psychobiology studies, we have found larger cortisol responses to waking in lower occupational grade groups both on working and non-working days in comparison with high status participants (Kunz-Ebrecht *et al.* 2004). We have recently studied socio-economic differences in cortisol responses to waking in a sample of older men and women living in the community, in order to determine whether differences are also present in people who are no longer working. This analysis involved 81 participants aged 65–80 years old, recruited from primary care health centres, and with no record of coronary heart disease, tachycardia, aortic valve regurgitation, dementia, psychosis, or cancer evident over the past five years. Saliva samples were taken on waking and then 10, 20, 30 and 60 minutes after waking up. Socio-economic position could not be measured by occupation, since participants were retired and some had never been in paid employment. Educational attainment was used as one indicator, but may not be completely satisfactory since education is typically completed early in life and may not reflect later experience. We therefore also assessed subjective social status with the single item measure developed by Adler *et al.* (2000). Participants were shown a ladder with 10 rungs, and were told that at the top of the ladder are the people who are best off – those with the most money, most education and best jobs. At the bottom are the people who are the worst off, and have the least money, least education and the worst jobs or no jobs. They were asked to place themselves on the rung on which they felt that they stood. Singh-Manoux *et al.* (2003) have shown that only 49 per cent of the variance of subjective social status in the Whitehall II cohort was accounted for by objective indicators such as employment grade, education, material deprivation and household income, suggesting that it may be assessing distinctive aspects of social position.

In our analyses of the cortisol response to waking, subjective social status rather than education emerged as having more consistent effects in this elderly sample (Wright and Steptoe 2005). Cortisol levels on waking did not vary with social status. Both higher and lower status participants showed increases after waking, but the rise was significantly greater in the lower social status group after controlling for gender, body mass index, waist/hip ratio, smoking status and time of waking. The increase was some 80 per cent larger in the lower status group.

These results are cross-sectional and their significance for health has not yet been directly demonstrated. Nevertheless, the findings that are beginning to emerge from naturalistic physiological monitoring studies suggest that lower socio-economic position is characterized by moderate disturbances of biological function that may in turn contribute to increased risk of physical disease.

Conclusions and future directions

Several exciting findings relating socio-economic position with biological responses have emerged in recent years. Nevertheless, this research field is still in its infancy. Most findings are cross-sectional, and do not conclusively demonstrate that disturbances of psychobiological responsivity mediate the socio-economic gradient in disease risk. Prospective studies are urgently needed, as are investigations that include measures of subclinical disease such as carotid IMT and plaque. If psychobiological pathways are indeed relevant, it is important to discover how much of the variance in disease risk they carry. We would like to know exactly how influential these processes are in comparison with behavioural and other pathways. This knowledge will help to determine whether treatments or preventive measures that address psychobiological processes (such as stress management or pharmacological methods) could ultimately prove valuable in the public health context.

These are issues for the future, and it is to be hoped that the present generation of studies will be superseded by investigations that have greater statistical power, and are more sophisticated from both the psychosocial and biological perspectives. Psychobiological studies hold great promise in helping to explain socio-economic gradients in health and disease risk, and the present findings must encourage more vigorous efforts to understand these processes.

References

Abbott DH, Keverne EB, Bercovitch FB *et al.* (2003). Are subordinates always stressed? A comparative analysis of rank differences in cortisol levels among primates. *Hormones and Behavior*, **43**, 67–82.

Adam EK and Gunnar MR (2001). Relationship functioning and home and work demands predict individual differences in diurnal cortisol patterns in women. *Psychoneuroendocrinology*, **26**, 189–208.

Adler NE, Epel ES, Castellazzo G and Ickovics JR (2000). Relationship of subjective and objective social status with psychological and physiological functioning: preliminary data in healthy white women. *Health Psychology*, **19**, 586–92.

Baker B, Helmers K, O'Kelly B, Sakinofsky I, Abelsohn A and Tobe S (1999). Marital cohesion and ambulatory blood pressure in early hypertension. *American Journal of Hypertension*, **12**, 227–30.

Barnes VA, Treiber FA, Musante L, Turner JR, Davis H and Strong WB (2000). Ethnicity and socio-economic status: impact on cardiovascular activity at rest and during stress in youth with a family history of hypertension. *Ethnicity & Disease*, **10**, 4–16.

Barnett RC, Steptoe A and Gareis KC (2005). Marital-role quality and stress-related psychobiological indicators. *Annals of Behavioral Medicine*. **30**, 36–43.

Bateson P and Bradshaw EL (1997). Physiological effects of hunting red deer (*Cervus elaphus*). *Proceedings of the Royal Society of London, Series B: Biological Sciences*, **264**, 1707–14.

Blumenthal JA, Thyrum ET and Siegel WC (1995). Contribution of job strain, job status and marital status to laboratory and ambulatory blood pressure in patients with mild hypertension. *Journal of Psychosomatic Research*, **39**, 133–44.

Brandtstadter J, Baltes-Gotz B, Kirschbaum C and Hellhammer D (1991). Developmental and personality correlates of adrenocortical activity as indexed by salivary cortisol: observations in the age range of 35 to 65 years. *Journal of Psychosomatic Research*, **35**, 173–85.

Brydon L, Edwards S, Jia H et al. (2005). Psychological stress increases interleukin-1 beta gene expression in human mononuclear cells. *Brain, Behavior, and Immunity.* **19**, 540–6.

Brydon L, Edwards S, Mohamed-Ali V and Steptoe A (2004). Socio-economic status and stress-induced increases in interleukin-6. *Brain, Behavior, and Immunity*, **18**, 281–90.

Brydon L and Steptoe A (2005). Stress-induced increases in interleukin-6 and fibrinogen predict ambulatory blood pressure at 3-year follow up. *Journal of Hypertension*, **23**, 1001–7.

Carroll D, Davey Smith G, Sheffield D, Shipley MJ and Marmot MG (1997). The relationship between socio-economic status, hostility, and blood pressure reactions to mental stress in men: data from the Whitehall II study. *Health Psychology*, **16**, 131–6.

Carroll D, Harrison LK, Johnston DW et al. (2000). Cardiovascular reactions to psychological stress: the influence of demographic variables. *Journal of Epidemiology and Community Health*, **54**, 876–7.

Cavelaars AEJM, Kunst AE and Mackenbach JP (1997). Socio-economic differences in risk factors for morbidity and mortality in the European Community. *Journal of Health Psychology*, **2**, 353–72.

Cohen S, Line S, Manuck SB, Rabin BS, Heise ER and Kaplan JR (1997). Chronic social stress, social status, and susceptibility to upper respiratory infections in nonhuman primates. *Psychosomatic Medicine*, **59**, 213–21.

Costa M, Steptoe A, Cropley M and Griffith J (1999). Ambulatory blood pressure monitoring is associated with reduced physical activity during everyday life. *Psychosomatic Medicine*, **61**, 806–11.

Danesh J, Collins R, Peto R and Lowe GD (2000). Haematocrit, viscosity, erythrocyte sedimentation rate: meta-analyses of prospective studies of coronary heart disease. *European Heart Journal*, **21**, 515–20.

Davies MJ (1996). Stability and instability: two faces of coronary atherosclerosis. The Paul Dudley White Lecture 1995. *Circulation*, **94**, 2013–20.

Dekker JM, Crow RS, Folsom AR et al. (2000). Low heart rate variability in a 2-minute rhythm strip predicts risk of coronary heart disease and mortality from several causes: the ARIC Study (Atherosclerosis Risk In Communities). *Circulation*, **102**, 1239–44.

Dickerson SS and Kemeny ME (2004). Acute stressors and cortisol responses: a theoretical integration and synthesis of laboratory research. *Psychological Bulletin*, **130**, 355–91.

Dowler E (2001). Inequalities in diet and physical activity in Europe. *Public Health Nutrition*, **4**, 701–9.

Egeland GM, Burkhart GA, Schnorr TM, Hornung RW, Fajen JM and Lee ST (1992). Effects of exposure to carbon disulphide on low density lipoprotein cholesterol concentration and diastolic blood pressure. *British Journal of Industrial Medicine*, **49**, 287–93.

Evans P, Der G, Ford G, Hucklebridge F, Hunt K and Lambert S (2000). Social class, sex, and age differences in mucosal immunity in a large community sample. *Brain, Behavior, and Immunity*, **14**, 41–8.

Gump BB and Matthews K (1999). Do background stressors influence reactivity to and recovery from acute stressors? *Journal of Applied Social Psychology*, **29**, 469–94.

Gump BB, Matthews KA and Raikkonen K (1999). Modeling relationships among socio-economic status, hostility, cardiovascular reactivity, and left ventricular mass in African-American and White children. *Health Psychology*, **18**, 140–50.

Hellhammer DH, Buchtal J, Gutberlet I and Kirschbaum C (1997). Social hierarchy and adrenocortical stress reactivity in men. *Psychoneuroendocrinology*, 22, 643–50.

Henry JP and Stephens PM (1977). *Stress, health, and the social environment.* Springer-Verlag, New York.

Henry JP, Stephens PM and Santisteban GA (1975). A model of psychosocial hypertension showing reversibility and progression of cardiovascular complications. *Circulation Research*, 36, 156–64.

Hulshof KF, Brussaard JH, Kruizinga AG, Telman J and Lowik MR (2003). Socio-economic status, dietary intake and 10 y trends: the Dutch National Food Consumption Survey. *European Journal of Clinical Nutrition*, 57, 128–37.

Jayo JM, Shively CA, Kaplan JR and Manuck SB (1993). Effects of exercise and stress on body fat distribution in male cynomolgus monkeys. *International Journal of Obesity and Related Metabolic Disorders*, 17, 597–604.

Jennings JR, Kamarck TW, Everson-Rose SA, Kaplan GA, Manuck SB and Salonen JT (2004). Exaggerated blood pressure responses during mental stress are prospectively related to enhanced carotid atherosclerosis in middle-aged Finnish men. *Circulation*, 110, 2198–203.

Kamarck TW, Shiffman S, Smithline L *et al.* (1998). Effects of task strain, social conflict, and emotional activation on ambulatory cardiovascular activity: daily life consequences of recurring stress in a multiethnic adult sample. *Health Psychology*, 17, 17–29.

Kaplan JR and Manuck SB (1999). Status, stress, and atherosclerosis: the role of environment and individual behavior. *Annals of the New York Academy of Sciences*, 896, 145–61.

Kaplan JR, Manuck SB, Clarkson TB, Lusso FM, Taub DM and Miller EW (1983). Social stress and atherosclerosis in normocholesterolemic monkeys. *Science*, 220, 733–5.

Kapuku GL, Treiber FA and Davis HC (2002). Relationships among socio-economic status, stress induced changes in cortisol, and blood pressure in African-American males. *Annals of Behavioral Medicine*, 24, 320–5.

Kiechl S, Egger G, Mayr M *et al.* (2001). Chronic infections and the risk of carotid atherosclerosis: prospective results from a large population study. *Circulation*, 103, 1064–70.

King AC, Oka RK and Young DR (1994). Ambulatory blood pressure and heart rate responses to the stress of work and caregiving in older women. *Journal of Gerontology*, 49, M239–45.

Kirschbaum C and Hellhammer DH (2000). Salivary cortisol. In: Fink G (ed.) *Encyclopedia of stress, Vol 3*, pp. 379–83. Academic Press, San Diego, CA.

Kristenson M, Kucinskiene Z, Bergdahl B and Orth-Gomer K (2001). Risk factors for coronary heart disease in different socio-economic groups of Lithuania and Sweden – the LiVicordia Study. *Scandinavian Journal of Public Health*, 29, 140–50.

Kudielka BM and Kirschbaum C (2003). Awakening cortisol responses are influenced by health status and awakening time but not by menstrual cycle phase. *Psychoneuroendocrinology*, 28, 35–47.

Kunz-Ebrecht SR, Kirschbaum C, Marmot M and Steptoe A (2004). Differences in cortisol awakening response on work days and weekends in women and men from the Whitehall II cohort. *Psychoneuroendocrinology*, 29, 516–28.

Kunz-Ebrecht SR, Mohamed-Ali V, Feldman PJ, Kirschbaum C and Steptoe A (2003). Cortisol responses to mild psychological stress are inversely associated with proinflammatory cytokines. *Brain, Behavior, and Immunity*, 17, 373–83.

Landsbergis PA, Schnall PL, Pickering TG, Warren K and Schwartz JE (2003). Lower socio-economic status among men in relation to the association between job strain and blood pressure. *Scandinavian Journal of Work, Environment and Health*, **29**, 206–15.

Lantz PM, Lynch JW, House JS *et al.* (2001). Socio-economic disparities in health change in a longitudinal study of US adults: the role of health-risk behaviors. *Social Science and Medicine*, **53**, 29–40.

Laukkanen JA, Kurl S, Salonen R, Lakka TA, Rauramaa R and Salonen JT (2004). Systolic blood pressure during recovery from exercise and the risk of acute myocardial infarction in middle-aged men. *Hypertension*, **44**, 820–5.

Light KC, Brownley KA, Turner JR *et al.* (1995). Job status and high-effort coping influence work blood pressure in women and blacks. *Hypertension*, **25**, 554–9.

Lovallo WR (2004). *Stress and health: biological and psychological interactions*, 2nd edn. Sage, Thousand Oaks, CA.

Lupien SJ, King S, Meaney MJ and McEwen BS (2000). Child's stress hormone levels correlate with mother's socio-economic status and depressive state. *Biological Psychiatry*, **48**, 976–80.

Lusis AJ (2000). Atherosclerosis. *Nature*, **407**, 233–41.

Lynch JW, Everson SA, Kaplan GA, Salonen R and Salonen JT (1998). Does low socio-economic status potentiate the effects of heightened cardiovascular responses to stress on the progression of carotid atherosclerosis? *American Journal of Public Health*, **88**, 389–94.

Manuck SB, Kaplan JR and Clarkson TB (1983). Behaviorally induced heart rate reactivity and atherosclerosis in cynomolgus monkeys. *Psychosomatic Medicine*, **45**, 95–102.

Marmot MG, Davey Smith G, Stansfeld S *et al.* (1991). Health inequalities among British civil servants: the Whitehall II study. *Lancet*, **337**, 1387–93.

Matthews KA, Raikkonen K, Everson SA *et al.* (2000). Do the daily experiences of healthy men and women vary according to occupational prestige and work strain? *Psychosomatic Medicine*, **62**, 346–53.

McEwen BS (1998). Protective and damaging effects of stress mediators. *New England Journal of Medicine*, **338**, 171–9.

McEwen BS (2003). Mood disorders and allostatic load. *Biological Psychiatry*, **54**, 200–7.

McEwen BS and Seeman T (1999). Protective and damaging effects of mediators of stress: elaborating and testing the concepts of allostasis and allostatic load. *Annals of the New York Academy of Sciences*, **896**, 30–47.

Michelson AD, Barnard MR, Krueger LA, Valeri CR and Furman MI (2001). Circulating monocyte-platelet aggregates are a more sensitive marker of *in vivo* platelet activation than platelet surface P-selectin: studies in baboons, human coronary intervention, and human acute myocardial infarction. *Circulation*, **104**, 1533–7.

Miller TQ, Smith TW, Turner CW, Guijarro ML and Hallet AJ (1996). A meta-analytic review of research on hostility and physical health. *Psychological Bulletin*, **119**, 322–48.

Mirowsky J and Ross CE (2003). *Social causes of psychological distress*, 2nd edn. Aldine De Gruyter, New York.

Owen N, Poulton T, Hay FC, Mohamed-Ali V and Steptoe A (2003). Socio-economic status, C-reactive protein, immune factors, and responses to acute mental stress. *Brain, Behavior, and Immunity*, **17**, 286–95.

Owens JF, Stoney CM and Matthews KA (1993). Menopausal status influences ambulatory blood pressure levels and blood pressure changes during mental stress. *Circulation*, **88**, 2794–802.

Pruessner JC, Wolf OT, Hellhammer DH *et al.* (1997). Free cortisol levels after awakening: a reliable biological marker for the assessment of adrenocortical activity. *Life Sciences*, **61**, 2539–49.

Pruessner M, Hellhammer DH, Pruessner JC and Lupien SJ (2003). Self-reported depressive symptoms and stress levels in healthy young men: associations with the cortisol response to awakening. *Psychosomatic Medicine*, **65**, 92–9.

Raison CL and Miller AH (2003). When not enough is too much: the role of insufficient glucocorticoid signaling in the pathophysiology of stress-related disorders. *American Journal of Psychiatry*, **160**, 1554–65.

Roberts AD, Wessely S, Chalder T, Papadopoulos A and Cleare AJ (2004). Salivary cortisol response to awakening in chronic fatigue syndrome. *British Journal of Psychiatry*, **184**, 136–41.

Rose KM, North K, Arnett DK *et al.* (2004). Blood pressure and pulse responses to three stressors: associations with sociodemographic characteristics and cardiovascular risk factors. *Journal of Human Hypertension*, **18**, 333–41.

Rosmond R and Bjorntorp P (2000). Occupational status, cortisol secretory pattern, and visceral obesity in middle-aged men. *Obesity Research*, **8**, 445–50.

Ross R (1999). Atherosclerosis – an inflammatory disease. *New England Journal of Medicine*, **340**, 115–26.

Sapolsky RM (1990). A. E. Bennett Award paper. Adrenocortical function, social rank, and personality among wild baboons. *Biological Psychiatry*, **28**, 862–78.

Schlotz W, Hellhammer J, Schulz P and Stone AA (2004). Perceived work overload and chronic worrying predict weekend-weekday differences in the cortisol awakening response. *Psychosomatic Medicine*, **66**, 207–14.

Schnall PL, Landsbergis PA and Baker D (1994). Job strain and cardiovascular disease. *Annual Review of Public Health*, **15**, 381–411.

Schrijvers CT, Stronks K, van de Mheen HD and Mackenbach JP (1999). Explaining educational differences in mortality: the role of behavioral and material factors. *American Journal of Public Health*, **89**, 535–40.

Schuler JL and O'Brien WH (1997). Cardiovascular recovery from stress and hypertension risk factors: a meta-analytic review. *Psychophysiology*, **34**, 649–59.

Seckl JR, Morton NM, Chapman KE and Walker BR (2004). Glucocorticoids and 11beta-hydroxysteroid dehydrogenase in adipose tissue. *Recent Progress in Hormone Research*, **59**, 359–93.

Seeman TE, McEwen BS, Rowe JW and Singer BH (2001). Allostatic load as a marker of cumulative biological risk: MacArthur studies of successful aging. *Proceedings of the National Academy of Sciences of the United States of America*, **98**, 4770–5.

Shively CA and Clarkson TB (1994). Social stress and coronary artery atherosclerosis in female monkeys. *Arteriosclerosis, Thrombosis, and Vascular Biology*, **14**, 721–6.

Siegrist J, Klein D and Voigt K-H (1997). Linking sociological with physiological data: the model of effort-reward imbalance at work. *Acta Physiologica Scandinavica*, **161**, Suppl **640**, 112–16.

Singer MT (1974). Engagement-involvement: a central phenomenon in psychophysiological research. *Psychosomatic Medicine*, **36**, 1–17.

Singh-Manoux A, Adler NE and Marmot MG (2003). Subjective social status: its determinants and its association with measures of ill-health in the Whitehall II study. *Social Science and Medicine*, **56**, 1321–33.

Smeeth L, Thomas SL, Hall AJ, Hubbard R, Farrington P and Vallance P (2004). Risk of myocardial infarction and stroke after acute infection or vaccination. *New England Journal of Medicine*, **351**, 2611–8.

Steptoe A (1985). Theoretical bases for task selection in cardiovascular psychophysiology. In: A Steptoe, H Ruddel and H Neus (eds) *Clinical and methodological issues in cardiovascular psychophysiology*, pp. 6–15. Springer-Verlag, Berlin.

Steptoe A and Ayers S (2004). Stress, health and illness. In: S Sutton, A Baum, M Johnston (eds) *Sage handbook of health psychology*, pp. 169–96. Sage, London.

Steptoe A and Brydon L (2005). Associations between acute lipid stress responses and fasting lipid levels three years later. *Health Psychology*, **24**, 601–607.

Steptoe A, Cropley M, Griffith J and Kirschbaum C (2000). Job strain and anger expression predict early morning elevations in salivary cortisol. *Psychosomatic Medicine*, **62**, 286–92.

Steptoe A, Feldman PM, Kunz S, Owen N, Willemsen G and Marmot M (2002). Stress responsivity and socio-economic status: a mechanism for increased cardiovascular disease risk? *European Heart Journal*, **23**, 1757–63.

Steptoe A, Fieldman G, Evans O and Perry L (1993). Control over work pace, job strain and cardiovascular responses in middle-aged men. *Journal of Hypertension*, **11**, 751–9.

Steptoe A, Kunz-Ebrecht S, Owen N *et al.* (2003a). Influence of socio-economic status and job control on plasma fibrinogen responses to acute mental stress. *Psychosomatic Medicine*, **65**, 137–44.

Steptoe A, Kunz-Ebrecht S, Owen N *et al.* (2003b). Socio-economic status and stress-related biological responses over the working day. *Psychosomatic Medicine*, **65**, 461–70.

Steptoe A, Kunz-Ebrecht S, Rumley A and Lowe GD (2003c). Prolonged elevations in haemostatic and rheological responses following psychological stress in low socio-economic status men and women. *Thrombosis and Haemostasis*, **89**, 83–90.

Steptoe A, Magid K, Edwards S, Brydon L, Hong Y and Erusalimsky J (2003d). The influence of psychological stress and socio-economic status on platelet activation in men. *Atherosclerosis*, **168**, 57–63.

Steptoe A and Marmot M (2005a). Impaired cardiovascular recovery following stress predicts 3 year increases in blood pressure. *Journal of Hypertension*, **23**, 529–36.

Steptoe A and Marmot M (2005b). Socio-economic position and coronary heart disease: a psychobiological perspective. In: LJ Waite (ed.) *Aging, health, and public policy*, pp. 133–50. Population Council, New York.

Steptoe A, Owen N, Kunz-Ebrecht S and Brydon L (2004a). Loneliness and neuroendocrine, cardiovascular, and inflammatory stress responses in middle-aged men and women. *Psychoneuroendocrinology*, **29**, 593–611.

Steptoe A, Siegrist J, Kirschbaum C and Marmot M (2004b). Effort–reward imbalance, overcommitment, and measures of cortisol and blood pressure over the working day. *Psychosomatic Medicine*, **66**, 323–9.

Steptoe A and Vögele C (1991). The methodology of mental stress testing in cardiovascular research. *Circulation*, **83**, II14–II24.

Sterling P and Eyer J (1988). Allostasis: a new paradigm to explain arousal pathology. In: S Fisher and J Reason (eds) *Handbook of life stress, cognition and health*, pp. 629–49. John Wiley, New York.

Treiber FA, Kamarck T, Schneiderman N, Sheffield D, Kapuku G and Taylor T (2003). Cardiovascular reactivity and development of preclinical and clinical disease states. *Psychosomatic Medicine*, **65**, 46–62.

Turner RJ, Wheaton B and Lloyd DA (1995). The epidemiology of social stress. *American Sociological Revue*, **60**, 104–25.

Uchino BN, Cacioppo JT and Kiecolt-Glaser JK (1996). The relationship between social support and physiological processes: a review with emphasis on underlying mechanisms and implications for health. *Psycholical Bulletin*, **119**, 488–531.

Van Cauter E, Leproult R and Plat L (2000). Age-related changes in slow wave sleep and REM sleep and relationship with growth hormone and cortisol levels in healthy men. *Journal of the American Medical Association*, **284**, 861–8.

van Eck M, Berkhof H, Nicolson N and Sulon J (1996). The effects of perceived stress, traits, mood states, and stressful daily events on salivary cortisol. *Psychosomatic Medicine*, **58**, 447–58.

Van Lenthe FJ, Gevers E, Joung IM, Bosma H and Mackenbach JP (2002). Material and behavioral factors in the explanation of educational differences in incidence of acute myocardial infarction: the Globe study. *Annals of Epidemiology*, **12**, 535–42.

Verdecchia P (2000). Prognostic value of ambulatory blood pressure: current evidence and clinical implications. *Hypertension*, **35**, 844–51.

Vrijkotte TG, van Doornen LJ and de Geus EJ (2000). Effects of work stress on ambulatory blood pressure, heart rate, and heart rate variability. *Hypertension*, **35**, 880–6.

Wardle J, Farrell M, Hillsdon M, Jarivs M, Sutton S and Thorogood M (1999). Smoking, drinking, physical activity and screening uptake and health inequalities. In: D Gordon, M Shaw, D Dorling and G Davey Smith (eds) *Inequalities in health*, pp. 213–39. Policy Press, Bristol.

Weiner H (1992). *Perturbing the organism: the biology of stressful experience*. University of Chicago Press, Chicago, IL.

Williams JK, Kaplan JR and Manuck SB (1993). Effects of psychosocial stress on endothelium-mediated dilation of atherosclerotic arteries in cynomolgus monkeys. *Journal of Clinical Investigation*, **92**, 1819–23.

Wilson DK, Kliewer W, Plybon L and Sica DA (2000). Socio-economic status and blood pressure reactivity in healthy black adolescents. *Hypertension*, **35**, 496–500.

Wright CE and Steptoe A (2005). Subjective socio-economic position, gender and cortisol responses to waking in an elderly population. *Psychoneuroendocrinology*, **30**, 582–90.

Chapter 6

Socio-economic position and health: the role of coping

Margareta Kristenson

Introduction

People with low socio-economic status (SES) have poorer prospects for health compared to people with high socio-economic status. This chapter explores the hypothesis that personal psychosocial resources are important mediators for these effects. In particular, coping ability, i.e. the individual's capacity to cope with life circumstances, will be assessed as a possible pathway. First, a presentation will be made on different concepts embracing the availability of personal psychosocial resources and the theoretical background for stating that these factors may mediate socio-economic effects on health will be reviewed. In a next step, possible psychobiological mechanisms will be explored and some recent empirical data supporting these assumptions are presented. Finally, implications for interventions will be discussed in relation to whether intervention on psychological factors is desirable, possible or even necessary if the aim is to reduce negative health effects of low SES.

Socio-economic status and health

Possible causes for socio-economic differences in health

Several possible causes for socio-economic differences in health have been explored in the literature. Genetic characteristics define the individual risk for disease, thereby also influencing people's life chances and social mobility, but genetic factors cannot explain differences in health between larger populations, which have developed over short time periods (Marmot and Wilkinson 1999). Social mobility does contribute to socio-economic differences in health, but only modestly, and the causal pathway from social status to health is stronger than the reverse. Socio-economic differences in health are not merely a result of selective social mobility: rather social structure has an impact on health status (Mulato and Schooler 2002). People with low SES tend to use health services to a lesser extent, which may affect disability and well-being, but these differences have not contributed to explaining socio-economic differences in health status (van Lenthe *et al.* 2004). Negative lifestyle factors, such as smoking, low physical activity in leisure time and excessive alcohol intake are more prevalent among people with low socio-economic status, and lifestyle factors explain about 25 per cent of the variance in scores of socio-economic differences in health. However, choices of lifestyle are not freely chosen but are dependent on both structural and psychosocial factors (Lantz *et al.* 1998). Finally, psychosocial factors are unevenly distributed between social classes and have been demonstrated to influence the SES–health relationship (Taylor and Seeman 1999).

Some characteristics of socio-economic differences in health

The findings that people with low SES tend to suffer from worse health are seen for several measures of social status, for example for education, occupation and income. These variables are interrelated, but represent different dimensions of social inequality. Education relates more to social status in early life as compared to present occupation, which defines adult social status. Income, in turn, describes availability of material resources but also a level of prestige (Marmot and Wilkinson 1999). The parallel relations to health, which have been demonstrated for these different measures of social status, suggest that research needs to be carried out into the mechanisms, which are common to these three states. An underlying domain may exist behind traditional measures of socio-economic position. Common for these states is a potential for social dominance and power. Moreover, individual's perception about the magnitude of their power and control over their own lives seems to be important for social differentials in health. This suggestion is supported by findings that, compared to objective indicators, subjective social status was more consistently and strongly related to psychological and physiological function (Adler *et al.* 2000). It is also supported by the repeated finding of a gradient across the social spectrum, rather than a threshold effect, suggesting that it is the position within the social hierarchy that is important for health (Marmot and Wilkinson 1999). Moreover, socio-economic differences in health are shown for a wide range of diseases and health problems, i.e. coronary heart disease (CHD), diabetes, gastrointestinal disease, respiratory diseases, arthritis, as well as for adverse birth outcomes, accidents and violent deaths (van Lenthe *et al.* 2004). This indicates that we should not look for risk factors which are specific for single groups of defined diseases but rather look for causes which have more general effects. One possible mechanism is through general susceptibility (Marmot *et al.* 1984). This term, sometimes regarded as 'mystic miasma' can, using today's knowledge on psychoneuroendocrinology and psychoneuroimmunology, be traced to fundamental stress mechanisms on cellular and subcellular levels (McEwen 2000). Thus, one question is whether stress – or rather resilience to stress – is important for socio-economic differences in health. This text will not focus on stress exposure but on individual characteristics, i.e. how people's perception of and attitudes toward stress exposure affect their health. This may be different depending on their social standing.

Coping and related concepts

A frame of reference

Over the years coping has acquired a variety of conceptual meanings. Being commonly used interchanging with such kindred concepts as mastery, defence and adaptation, the coping concept has become an umbrella term covering different theoretical approaches, measurements and interpretations such as strategies, profiles or expectations. Because of its multiple meaning it is necessary to specify one's own working definition. Pearlin and Schooler suggested that coping should be used to refer to as 'any response to external life strains that serves to prevent, avoid or control emotional distress. This is inseparable both from the life-strains experienced by people and from the state of their inner emotional life' (Pearlin and Schooler 1978). Thus, according to this definition, coping must be examined in relation to, on one hand, the problems which people encounter in the social environment and, on the other, the potential emotional impact of these problems. Pearlin and Schooler also suggested a distinction between three kinds of resources that are important for the emotional impact of social strain: social resources, psychological resources (coping ability) and specific coping responses (coping strategies).

Social environment

The most prominent research on stress exposure and health has been done according to characteristics of the work environment, while fewer studies have focused on family life and other parts of life outside work. The main theoretical models on psychosocial work environment build on an interaction between work exposure and individual perception of this exposure. The demand–control (job strain) model states that health depends on the interaction between experienced demands and the perceived feeling of control and 'decision latitude' over work, and the latter has shown the strongest effects on health development. The concept of decision latitude contains two dimensions: intellectual discretion (learning opportunities) and authority over decision, and research has demonstrated that both these domains are important factors for health development (Karasek and Theorell 1990).

The Siegrist model of effort/reward imbalance focuses on the balance between efforts made and perceived rewards, such as esteem, salary, promotions and job security. In this model, two sources for high effort at work have been defined: an extrinsic source; the demands on the job, and an intrinsic source; the motivations of the individual in a demanding situation. In the latter regard, the concept 'overcommitment' was introduced as a personal pattern of coping with the demands at work. It identifies individuals with an intrinsic need of exaggerated work-related efforts that may not be balanced by available rewards (Siegrist 2002). Both job strain and effort–reward imbalance are unequally distributed, both between and within societies, and both models have, in prospective studies, predicted all-cause and CHD death (Marmot and Wilkinson 1999) (see also Chapter 4).

Social resources

In addition to the potential stress from exposures in the social environment, this environment also provides resources. These social resources are represented in the interpersonal networks of which people are a part and which are potential sources of crucial support. Social support at work has been added to the Karasek and Theorell model, referring to perceived support from superiors and colleagues, and has been demonstrated to have a beneficial effect on health development (Marmot and Wilkinson 1999). Likewise, availability of social support in private life and social integration in wider social networks are well known as important determinants for health and have predicted lower risk for all cause mortality and for specific outcomes such as CHD and cancer. These social resources are, in several studies, found to be less prevalent among individuals with low SES (Mickelson and Kubzansky 2003) (see also Chapter 3).

Coping strategies and coping ability

In the distinction between social resources, psychological resources (coping ability) and specific coping responses (coping strategies), the first one, i.e. between social factors and 'coping', is well documented in the literature. In contrast, the distinction between coping *strategies* and coping *ability* is often less clear.

Coping *strategies* are the behaviours, cognitions and perceptions in which people engage when actually contending with life problems/situations (Pearlin and Schooler 1978). The main strategies include, on one hand, responses that modify the situation (problem-focused strategies, instrumental, mastery-oriented or active coping) and, on the other hand, responses that function to control the meaning of the situation by cognitively neutralizing the threat or aiming at managing the stress (emotion-focused or 'passive' coping).

Coping *ability* means personality characteristics that people draw upon to meet new demands and changes in their environment. These resources, residing within the self, can be fundamental barriers to the stressful consequences of social strain. Pearlin and Schooler identified three kinds of resources. The first two are closely related but according to empirical data, independent: 'self-esteem' refers to the positiveness of one's attitude towards one self while 'self-denigration' refers to negative attitudes towards oneself. The third dimension is called 'mastery' and means the extent to which one regards one's life chances as being under one's own control in contrast to being fatalistically ruled (Pearlin and Schooler 1978). Pearlin *et al.* developed an instrument for these three dimensions. The scale of mastery is commonly used and often under the term 'coping' (meaning coping ability). The items in the scale of mastery include 'I have no way to solve important things in my life', 'I often feel helpless in dealing with problems of my life', 'I sometimes feel pushed around in life', 'What happens in the future mostly depends on me', 'I can do about anything I really set my mind to do'. As can be seen, the questions in this scale mainly refer to things related to individual's personal life. In the following text we shall focus on coping ability and related concepts.

Expectancies, learning and coping

Levine and Ursin have developed a more dynamic approach to the coping concept. They define coping as 'positive outcome expectancy, based on earlier experiences on the interaction between the exposure and the response to this exposure'. The acquisition of this expectancy is based on the interaction between the exposure and the connected response (Ursin and Eriksen 2004). When the result is negative the individual stores this experience as negative outcome expectancy, and feels 'hopeless'. If the individual has learned that there is no relationship between their responses and the outcome, the individual develops 'helplessness'. When the individuals feel they can manage the situation, they cope and feel that they master the situation. Many of these expectancies represent learning that has occurred early in life, which in turn influences later learning (Ursin and Eriksen 2004).

Coping has also been represented by other terms such as control (e.g. perceived control and locus of control), self-efficacy, sense of coherence and toughness. Several of these concepts are grasping a common central core. However all have specific connotations (see Chapter 7).

Control and self-efficacy

The concept of 'control' has been used extensively in the literature. The different constructs relating to control are many, e.g. in a review in 1996 more than 100 terms were identified (Skinner 1996). They could be separated into two classes: actual control or the objective control conditions present in the context of the person, and perceived control, or the individual's beliefs about how much control is available.

Perceived control (also named personal control, sense of control or subjective control) relates to the extent to which agents perceive that they can intentionally produce desired outcomes and prevent undesired ones. Classical work on learned helplessness showed that prolonged exposure to situations with low actual control produces cognitive, motivational and emotional deficits, that is, they lead to low perceived control also in situations with high actual control (Skinner 1996). Locus of control, response–outcome expectancy, and explanatory style are concepts relating to where individuals place the role of the actor. Internal locus of control means that individuals can, themselves, take important actions over their lives while external locus of control and universal helplessness mean that this is not possible as the power over their life is outside their authority.

Bandura introduced the concept of self-efficacy referring to the expectation of one's own competencies. He differentiates between self-efficacy and outcome expectation. While the latter refers to the anticipation of results of one's own action the former refers to one's ability to perform a certain action. High levels of perceived efficacy enable a person to cope with confidence and high motivation (Skinner 1996).

Sense of coherence

This concept was developed by the sociologist Aaron Antonovsky whose starting point was socio-economic differences in health. Later he focused on 'an alternative central paradigm for stress research' (Antonovsky 1979). Using a salutogenic perspective where the outcome was general health and not specific disease, he identified people who reported a good self-rated health even when exposed to heavy environmental strain. The psychological characteristic, which was common for people in this group, was named 'Sense of Coherence'. He defined this state as

> a global orientation that expresses the extent to which one has a pervasive, enduring though dynamic, feeling of confidence that one's internal and external environments are predictable and that there is a high probability that things will work out as well as can reasonably be expected.

(Antonovsky 1979)

The three main dimensions in the sense of coherence concept cover the ability to define life events as less stressful (comprehensibility), to mobilize resources to deal with encountered stressors (manageability), and motivation, desire, and commitment to cope (meaningfulness).

More specifically, comprehensibility means that life is ordered, consistent and makes sense, with reference to the future it implies predictability. Open-ended situations are tolerable, as there is confidence that one can make sense of them. On the other extreme life is chaotic, accidental and cognitively un-understandable. Manageability means on one end of the scale a paranoid situation; 'they are after me, things always happen to me, always have and always will'. At the other end of the scale things do not 'happen'. Problems may arise but somehow one will be able to manage, to tolerate, via one's own resources or with the help of a legitimate authority such as God. If the worst happens, one can learn to live with the problem. This might imply a strong internal locus of control; but it can also be dependent on trust in external recourses (friends or the doctor/counsellor). The third domain, meaningfulness, means that one must care enough about what one does in life, about what goes on in one's life, to wish to engage in it. Life is seen as a challenge, not a burden, as worthy of commitment.

Toughness

The term 'toughness' was defined as 'a capacity for a positive performance in even complex tasks, for emotional stability and for immune enhancement'. Dienstbier argued that people who seek challenges do so because they have a capacity to perform, they expect energy, not tension, and, for these people the challenge leads to a positive arousal pattern, to energy and success (Dienstbier 1989). The opposite circle can be identified for those who avoid challenges. They do so because they have less capacity to perform. They expect tension, harm and loss, and the arousal pattern also leads to tension, and to failure. In parallel, these loops of challenge and success vs. strain and failure lead to effects on immune status and somatic health development. Thus, this concept entails a psychobiological component, and we shall come back to this concept later in the chapter.

Coping ability, a common core among psychological resources for health

As seen from the above, there is both an overlap of, but also differences between, different constructs describing general psychological resources of individuals. They describe feelings of mastery over one's own life, of positive outcome expectancy, perceived ability to exert control over one's life, a sense that life is coherent and an ability to see stressors as challenges, not as threats. A common core seems to be a feeling of power over our own life, of optimism and harmony. The concepts are, in several cases, discussed in terms of barriers to stress, sometimes called general resistance resources, and they have all been related to good prospects for a positive health development.

Coping: prevalence and consequences

Prevalence of coping ability

Effective coping strategies are unequally distributed in society with people in dominant positions – men, highly educated and affluent people – making greater use of the mechanisms leading to higher levels of coping ability (mastery) and better outcome expectancy (Pearlin and Schooler 1978, Ursin and Eriksen 2004). Lower scale scores of coping ability have been demonstrated among people with low socio-economic position, both within and between countries. In a study using three national data sets, convergent findings were obtained with significant differences in control beliefs by social status; those with low income reporting lower levels of mastery (Lachman and Weaver 1998). Likewise, in a large public health survey in south-east Sweden in 1999 people with low education had, across all ages, lower scale scores of coping ability in terms of mastery. Moreover, women had, compared to men, lower mean levels of coping ability. Stratifying for gender, differences between educational groups were more pronounced among women than among men and a significant interaction effect was seen (p = 0.02) illustrating a higher risk of low coping ability for the combination of being a woman and having low education (Sjögren and Kristenson 2006) (Figures 6.1 and 6.2).

Likewise, in a comparison between middle-aged Swedish men and Lithuanian men (with a fourfold higher risk of myocardial infarction), the latter group had lower scale scores of coping (mastery). Within the countries people with low SES had lower coping ability. This was, among Swedish men, seen for several measures of social status: i.e. for occupation, education and

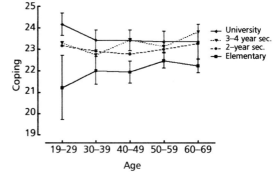

Figure 6.1 Mean scale scores on coping (mastery) in relation to education and age among men aged 25–69. N = 3355. ANOVA test of difference in coping between educational groups, adjusted for effect of age; p < 0.001.

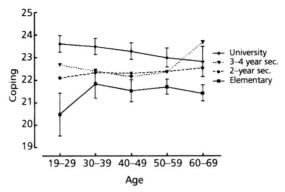

Figure 6.2 Mean scale scores on coping (mastery) in relation to education and age among women aged 25–69. N = 3884. ANOVA test of differences in coping between educational groups, adjusted for effect of age; p < 0.001.

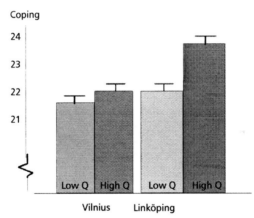

Figure 6.3 Mean scale scores on coping (mastery) in relation to income (highest vs. lowest income quartiles within the cities) among 50-year old men in Vilnius, Lithuania and Linköping, Sweden. N = 273. Test of linear regression of coping on income, adjusted for effect of residence; p = 0.003.

income (Figure 6.3), and, among both Swedish and Lithuanian men, also for decision latitude at work, which was used as a measure of occupational power (Kristenson *et al.* 2001).

Childhood, coping and socio-economic status

A coping child will learn that it does master new challenges and also learns to approach new and challenging tasks, since it expects success. Learning success (coping), or learning helplessness and hopelessness, will have a decisive influence on future learning (Kristenson *et al.* 2004) and to feelings of control over life. Socio-economic differences in health often have their origin in early life and the association between SES and health status can be detected already in childhood. In his first papers, Antonovsky claimed that sense of coherence would be stable after individuals had passed childhood. However, later research has challenged this view, and adult sense of coherence seems to be influenced by both individual conditions and societal changes also in adulthood.

Childhood socio-economic conditions also have effects on psychosocial characteristics in adulthood (van Lenthe *et al.* 2004) and these two factors, i.e. childhood SES and adult psychosocial status, appear to be complementary and additive risk factors for illness in adulthood (see Chapter 2).

Coping and mental health

Loss of coping or loss of availability of positive social interactions may thus lead to negative feelings. Starrin suggested that negative life events lead to feelings of shame, which can be so unbearable that we need to protect ourselves. This would lead to attacks against both others and self, to low self-esteem, less proneness to act, powerlessness and social isolation (Kristenson *et al.* 2004). In 1905 the Swedish novelist Hjalmar Söderberg described the 'pathway' from high self-esteem, via cynicism and social isolation to depression and hopelessness in a Swedish novel, *Doctor Glas.*

> You want to be loved,
> Failing that, to be admired,
> Failing that, to be feared,
> Failing that, to be loathed and despised.
> We need to affect others – somehow;
> The soul shudders at emptiness,
> And wants contact, whatever the price.

Empirical data on relations between coping (mastery) and individual characteristics also support this suggestion; with positive correlations to self-esteem ($r = 0.58$), and sense of coherence ($r = 0.56$,) and negative correlations to hostility ($r = -0.36$), depression ($r = -0.49$), vital exhaustion ($r = -0.55$) and hopelessness ($r = -0.66$), all p's < 0.001 (Kristenson 2004, Kristenson *et al.* 2004). Complementary to these cross-sectional data, a recent prospective study demonstrated that premorbid levels of mastery were significantly related to depressive symptoms one year after diagnosis of cardiac disease (van Jaarsveld *et al* 2005).

Socio-economic status, coping and health

Several studies have examined relations between SES, psychosocial factors and self-reported health outcomes. Using data from three cross-sectional, population-based, national surveys in 1993, 1994 and 1995 consistent results emerged demonstrating that high scale scores of depression were more prevalent among people with low income. At all income levels, higher coping ability (mastery) was related to better health and lower depression. Moreover, coping played a moderating role in the relation between income and depression; i.e. people with low income, who had high coping ability, had the same, low, level of depression as the high income group (Lachman and Weaver 1998). Using the 1994–1995 national population samples of Canadians, exposure to psychosocial stressors was tested as mediating mechanism for the social gradient in self-rated health. Higher exposure to stress, in terms of recent life events, was observed with decreasing income. Exposure to stress accounted for a significant part of the relationship between income and self-rated health and this was larger among men (26 per cent) than among women (6–15 per cent) (Orpana and Lemyre 2004). In a population-based sample of 3000 men from the US followed from 1974 to 1994 health was determined in terms of 'physical health condition that limits your activities', and psychosocial distress in terms of anxiety and 'self-deprecation' (feeling downcast or dejected). More than a third of the SES-health relationship was accounted for by the combined effect of lifestyle and psychosocial factors and the major part of this effect was seen from psychosocial factors (Mulato and Schooler 2002).

The validity of studies relating self-reported resources and self-reported outcomes could be questioned as correlations between psychological factors and self-reported health may be merely a reflection of an overlap between measures, and results be depending on a common factor such as neuroticism. However, evidence from US and Finnish studies show that both psychosocial factors and health behaviours account for some of the socio-economic gradient in health and effects were most pronounced at the lowest socio-economic levels (Cohen *et al.* 1999). Still, a more challenging question may be whether coping is also related to objective and 'hard' outcomes such as morbidity and death.

Coping and somatic disease

There is, today, an abundant literature on the effect of psychosocial risk factors on risk of somatic disease. This is the case both for factors in work and social environment and for individual characteristics. In the Kuopio study psychosocial factors in terms of depression, hopelessness, marital status, participation in social organizations and quality of social support were as strong as effects of lifestyle in explaining associations between income and mortality (all cause and cardiovascular) (Lynch *et al.* 1996).

There are also several studies, which have demonstrated effects of psychosocial resources on mortality: perceived control is a robust predictor of personal adjustment and success in a variety of life domains, such as coping (mastery), self-esteem and optimism, but also of mental and physical well-being and of all-cause mortality (Skinner 1996), and in a prospective study in the Netherlands perceived control explained a substantial part of socio-economic differences in mortality (van Lenthe *et al.* 2004) (see also Chapter 7 in this book). Sense of coherence has, in several studies, been related to lower risk of mortality, e.g. in a prospective study in United Kingdom 1996–2002 high scale scores of sense of coherence were associated with a 30 per cent reduction in mortality from all causes, cardiovascular disease and cancer, and this effect was independent of age, sex or prevalent chronic disease (Surtees *et al.* 2003).

High coping ability, using the measure of mastery, has been related to better health outcomes, both in terms of CHD prognosis after first myocardial infarction and of all-cause mortality. The latter was demonstrated in the Longitudinal Ageing Study Amsterdam where a large population sample of people aged 55–85 was followed over three years and social support, self-esteem, self-efficacy and coping (mastery) were assessed at baseline. After control for effects of lifestyle and illness, mastery was significantly related to risk of all-cause mortality. People with greater feelings of mastery had decreased risk of mortality; for each point of increase on the mastery scale the risk was reduced by OR = 0.93 (0.89–0.98) e.g. people scoring in the highest decile of the mastery scale had a 0.57-fold lower risk of dying compared to those in the lowest decile (Penninx *et al.* 1997).

Psychobiology

Stress, a possible pathway

We have discussed the theoretical basis and empirical data supporting the view that ability to cope with life is important not only for health but also in terms of somatic disease and death. One important question then arises: what are the possible pathways? Are findings effects of confounding, indirect effects of choices of lifestyle or other risk behaviour or is there a direct effect? We shall now explore the last hypothesis and look at stress mechanisms.

What is stress?

The word 'stress' is, in the literature, used with several connotations. It is used for (1) the *exposure* (stimulus, stressor), (2) the *experience of the situation* (self-reports), (3) the *stress response* (psycho-physiological activation or wakening response), and (4) the *experience of this somatic response* (self-reports). In this paper, the definition of the stress concept offered by Levine and Ursin (the stress response) is followed. This is a psychobiological concept, and should not be conceived of as either biological or psychological (Ursin and Eriksen 2004). The stress reaction, arousal (activation), is an adaptive response to exposure which is important both for positive health development and for survival. However, the same stress response may, if out of balance, be deleterious for health.

Cognitive activation theory

The Cognitive Activation Theory of Stress states that the stress response is identical to activation and should be regarded as a general alarm system (Ursin and Eriksen 2004). Activation (alarm) occurs whenever the organism registers that there is a discrepancy between what is expected (set value) and what really exists (actual value). This evaluation is dependent on cognitive processes evaluating the situation and the available resources, taking into account previous experience. This experience is stored as expectancies tied to the stimuli, and to the available responses. The theory builds on Activation Theory and is integrated with similar concepts from psychophysiology, psychoneuroendocrinology, and psychoneuroimmunology (Ursin and Eriksen 2004).

Psychobiology and allostasis

The general, non-specific activation response is characterized by increased wakefulness in the brain, increased metabolism and turnover of transmitters, increased muscle tone, specific behaviours, and vegetative, endocrine, and immune changes (Ursin and Eriksen 2004). The main components of the stress response are the hypothalamic–pituitary–adrenal axis (the HPA axis, with cortisol as main actor) the limbs of the autonomic nervous system (ANS) with the catecholamines adrenaline and noradrenaline and the immune system with interleukines as main biomarkers. These systems are closely interrelated. Cortisol is an important coordinator of the systems, i.e. one of the most important actions of cortisol seems to be to protect the body against self-defence systems so that they do not overreact and, themselves, damage the body (Munck, Guyre, and Holbrook, 1984).

Sterling and Eyer introduced the term 'allostasis' to illustrate that the organism must vary the parameters of the internal environment to match them appropriately to environmental demands. This requires continuous readjustment of all parameters toward new setpoints (Sterling and Eyer 1990).

McEwen has elaborated this concept to 'the process for actively maintaining homeostasis'. The systems, which vary according to demands, i.e. the HPA axis and ANS, actually help maintain those systems that are truly homeostatic, e.g. oxygen tension and pH. Thus allostasis is a better term for physiological coping mechanisms than homeostasis and a more comprehensive definition of allostasis is 'the process that keeps the organism alive and functioning' i.e. maintaining homeostasis or 'maintaining stability through change', and 'promoting adaptation and coping' (McEwen 2000).

Stress pathophysiology

While necessary for health and survival, stress reactions may also be harmful (McEwen 2000, Ursin and Eriksen 2004). Normally, these processes are controlled by precise feedback mechanisms. Pathology may occur if these mechanisms are overtaxed. McEwen uses the term 'allostatic load' to describe the 'wear and tear' and the 'chronic effects of non-adaptive reactions in changing environments' (McEwen 2000). Chronic elevations of hormones generally lead to downward regulation of receptors (Sterling and Eyer 1990) and, to obtain the same effect, a larger dose is needed. In parallel, no opportunities for relaxation may lead to loss of margins left for responding to additional challenges. Both changes may lead to organic pathology. The effects relate to metabolic disturbances such as insulin resistance, tissue damage in inflammation, infections and immunology, fluid loss, neurochemical activity and oxidative stress reactions. This loss of dynamic capacity to respond to, and to relax after, stress (loss of allostasis) could be a cause for the higher susceptibility to disease that has been found more often among individuals with low socio-economic status (Kristenson *et al.* 2004).

The hypothesis is based on the assumption that loss of allostasis is more common in individuals with low SES and on observations of lower levels of coping and personal control in the low compared to the high SES (Lachman and Weaver 1998, Taylor and Seeman 1999, Kristenson et al 2001). Coping leads to focused and *adequate responses*, followed by *relaxation* and *reduced* activation in man and animals while lack of coping, helplessness, and hopelessness lead to inability to relax, to sustained activation and a poorer capacity to respond to new challenges (Kristenson *et al.* 2004).

Psychoneuroendocrinology, psychosocial factors and the hypothalamic–pituitary–adrenal axis

Stress reactivity (response) can be evaluated using standardized laboratory stress testing or field studies e.g. ambulatory saliva sampling during an ordinary day. In both cases resting or baseline levels and stress responses are evaluated. The major part of research in this area has focused on relations between negative exposures (and risk factors) to stress reactivity, with less data on psychosocial resources. High stress exposures have been associated with higher stress reactivity of cortisol (McEwen 2000). However, in later stages of chronic stress recurrent high responsiveness seem to result in attenuated (reduced) cortisol reactivity and increased resting values (Sterling and Eyer 1990, McEwen 2000).

Using standardized laboratory stress testing several psychosocial risk factors have been related to reduced cortisol reactivity, e.g. men with effort–reward imbalance at work (Siegrist *et al.* 1997). Our group earlier reported an attenuated cortisol response to acute stress *and* raised baseline (resting) levels among middle-aged men who had unfavourable psychosocial characteristics (Kristenson *et al.* 2004). High vital exhaustion related to poor stress response while low scale scores on sense of coherence and coping were related to high baseline levels.

In several studies flattened diurnal slopes of saliva cortisol levels, i.e. smaller differences between morning and evening values, have been found among people exposed to chronic stress e.g. among middle-class mothers of two-year-old children with poor relationship functioning and high workload (Adam and Gunnar 2001). Also, prospective studies of cortisol reactivity have illustrated changes in reactivity over time. In a study of nurses and medical secretaries, exposed to dramatic organizational change, cortisol levels changed over time, with lower morning levels and higher levels in the evening after a period of long-term stress due to downsizing processes at the workplace (Hertting and Theorell 2002). In a parallel manner, cancer patients participating in a stress reduction programme reported lower stress levels after the intervention and their diurnal cortisol secretion patterns shifted towards a steeper decline (Carlsson *et al.* 2004). Moreover, a steep diurnal rhythm has been related to better prognosis among cancer patients and this has been demonstrated for both morbidity and mortality (Sephton *et al.* 2000).

Few studies have explicitly searched for effects of positive feelings on cortisol levels. A positive relationship between religiosity and mental health variables such as hope, optimism and sense of meaning in life, and physical health variables such as survival time has been demonstrated, and steeper diurnal slopes of cortisol were seen among fibromyalgia patients who were highly religious (Dedert *et al.* 2004). Also, a recent study examined people who were in love (defined as 'obsessively thinking about the partner more than four hours a day'). Couples who were in love had higher morning levels of cortisol compared to 'ordinary couples' (Marazziti and Canale 2004). The feelings involved in this state are, by most people, related to well-being, but also to a perceived capacity and ability to perform 'almost everything', i.e. very high coping ability.

Psychoneuroimmunology

Cytokines are protein substances, released by cells, that serve as intercellular signals to regulate the immune response to injury and infection (Kiecolt-Glaser *et al.* 2002). The signalling of cytokines is similar to classic hormones of the endocrine system and they can be characterized as communication molecules between immune cells and endothelial cells. Their key role is in the regulation of immune response and the coordination of the host response to infection. Cytokines can be classified in two basic classes based on their effect on the immune system, proinflammatory and anti-inflammatory. High levels of the pro-inflammatory cytokine interleukin-6 (IL-6) are related to higher risk of disease and death. IL-6 promotes the production of C-reactive protein, which is also an important predictor for myocardial infarction. IL-6 production is dependent on cortisol levels, but production of IL-6 can also be directly stimulated by negative emotions (hostility and depression) and stressful experiences (Kiecolt-Glaser *et al.* 2002). Few studies have explored relations between psychosocial resources and IL-6 levels, but high IL-6 levels were found among people with lack of job satisfaction and decision latitude (Theorell *et al.* 2000).

Socio-economic status and stress reactivity

In several animal studies, including primates, dominating males have *low resting* cortisol, high testosterone and high secondary sexual features in contrast to subordinate males (Kristenson *et al.* 2004). However, this is the case as long as hierarchies are stable, and when there is a change in the group, the dominant male has higher resting cortisol. There are few population-based human studies examining the role of social status on cortisol levels, but in a population sample of 767 individuals aged 35–65, high social status corresponded to higher morning cortisol levels (7–9 a.m.) i.e. to the arousal of awakening and a positive association between cortisol levels (morning) and indicators for successful development and personal well-being was observed (Brandstädter *et al.* 1991). The authors suggested that 'Life satisfaction and personal success was linked to a readiness to meet and capability to cope with novel and challenging situations.' Likewise, dominant soldiers had a stronger response to a new challenge compared to subordinates (Hellhammer *et al.* 1997) and in a study of 200 middle-aged men from Sweden and Lithuania, men with high status (similar for occupation, education and income) had lower baseline levels and stronger cortisol response to a standardized stress test (Kristenson *et al.* 2004). In the Whitehall study cortisol concentrations were higher among men with low socio-economic position, while among women, those with low position had lower cortisol levels over the day (Steptoe *et al.* 2003). Few studies have reported on IL-6 levels in relation to social status; but in laboratory stress-testing stress induced IL-6 levels were increased over prolonged times among people with low compared to those with high SES, suggesting that the former are less able to adapt to stress than the latter (Brydon *et al.* 2004).

Empirical data on socio-economic status, coping and biology

A health divide within Europe

In central and Eastern Europe a dramatic health decline has occurred during the last four decades. This development peaked in the transition period in the 1990s, when mean life expectancy was six years shorter compared to western Europe (Kristenson *et al.* 2004).

This was a period of dramatic social change, characterized by social disruption, economic hardship and low prospects for the future. More than half of the health decline was due to an increased mortality in CHD and in 1994 Lithuanian men had an approximately fourfold higher risk of myocardial death compared to Swedish men. The cause for this dramatic health divide within Europe has been debated. One suggestion is that it reflects socio-economic differences across the continent (Kristenson *et al.* 2004).

The LiVicordia study

In the cross sectional LiVicordia (Linköping Vilnius coronary artery disease assessment) study, performed 1993–1995, random samples of 150 middle-aged men in each of Vilnius, Lithuania and Linköping, Sweden, were compared. In addition to traditional risk factors for CHD a broad range of psychosocial and biological markers known to predict CHD, were tested. Traditional risk factors showed fairly small differences; systolic blood pressure was higher in Lithuanian men, smoking habits were similar, while cholesterol levels were higher in men from Sweden, and these factors could not explain the difference in risk of CHD between the countries. While having different drinking patterns, with more liquor and beer among Lithuanians and more wine among Swedes, there was no difference in total alcohol intake between the two groups (Kristenson *et al.* 2004).

In contrast, Lithuanian men had, on all measures tested, more unfavourable psychosocial characteristics. They reported higher job strain, lower social support at work, less emotional support and lower social integration than Swedish men. They also reported lower coping ability (mastery), lower self-esteem and lower sense of coherence, more overcomittment, more hostility, and higher scale scores of vital exhaustion (a state characterized by extended mental fatigue) and depression (Kristenson *et al.* 2004). A standardized laboratory stress test was also performed. This included a preparatory phase with relaxation and, at the end of this period, measures for resting (baseline) levels. Thereafter three stressors were presented; Anger recall, Mental arithmetic and the Cold pressor test. Serum and saliva samples were collected across and after the stress test period and analysed for cortisol. Lithuanian men had higher cortisol baseline levels and an attenuated cortisol response to the stressful situation. Low scale scores on coping (mastery) and sense of coherence were both correlated to high baseline cortisol, while poor cortisol responses was correlated to current smoking and high scale scores of vital exhaustion (Kristenson *et al.* 2004).

It has been suggested that east-west differences in health are caused by socio-economic differences across the continent. To test this hypothesis, a comparison was made of the prevalence of the above risk factors in high and low socio-economic groups within the two cities. Measures of social status were education, occupation, income and occupational power in terms of decision latitude at work. The same psychosocial characteristics that were found among Lithuanian men, as compared to Swedish men, were also found among men in low social classes within both cities, and this was the case for all four measures of social status: men with low SES had more job strain, lower scale scores of social integration, of coping and self-esteem, and higher vital exhaustion compared to men of high social class. They also had higher baseline cortisol, and a poorer cortisol response to a stressful situation (Kristenson *et al.* 2001).

The overall results indicate that difficulties with psychosocial life and negative expectations for the future are linked to an inadequate stress response. The higher baseline fits in with the sustained activation theory. One physiological possibility is that this stress response pattern represents a failure to turn off activation, but also, because of the heightened level of cortisol, an inability to turn on the responses to the adequate level needed. This fits with a state of sustained arousal leading to loss of dynamic capacity to respond to new challenges (Sterling and Eyer 1990, Kristenson *et al.* 2004).

The LinQuest study

In the LinQuest cross-sectional study, in the year 2000, 257 Swedish men and women aged 35–65 were investigated and psychosocial factors assessed via questionnaires. Cortisol reactivity was assessed via ambulatory saliva sampling.

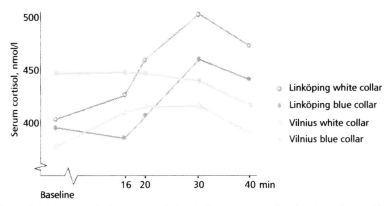

Figure 6.4 Mean cortisol serum levels in relation to occupation (white collar vs. blue collar) before and after a standardized laboratory stress test among 50-year old men in Vilnius, Lithuania and Linköping, Sweden. N = 183. Test of linear regression of serum cortisol on occupational status, adjusted for effect of residence p = 0.008 and p = 0.045 for baseline and deviation, respectively.

Saliva was collected at home at awakening, thirty minutes after awakening and in the evening. In partial correlations, after control for effects of confounders, diurnal deviation of cortisol levels was positively related to coping (mastery) and social support and negatively related to scale scores of cynicism, vital exhaustion and depression. Also, occupation was related to diurnal slope, with steeper slope related to higher status (Sjögren *et al.* 2005). Thus, in this study of ambulatory sampled saliva the same relations between psychosocial factors, social status and cortisol levels emerged as in the laboratory stress test.

In a subsample of 59 men and women IL-6 levels in serum and saliva were assessed and related to psychosocial factors. IL-6 levels were negatively related to coping and self-esteem and positively related to cynicism, hopelessness, vital exhaustion and depression (all $p < 0.05$) (Kristenson 2004). As can be seen, the same set of psychosocial factors were identified to be related to IL-6 as were related to cortisol, but with opposite signs; i.e. psychological resources were linked to low IL-6 levels and high cortisol reactivity with the opposite findings for psychosocial risk factors.

Implications for intervention

Synergistic effects of stress and lifestyle

Stressful social environments and low availability of protective resources are more common among people with low socio-economic status. Stress may affect health directly via the pathophysiological effects of loss of allostasis, or indirectly via lifestyle. People with low SES are known to have more unhealthy lifestyles, e.g. they eat more unhealthy food, smoke more and have more sedentary lifestyles. A major obstacle for the introduction, acceptance, and compliance with new rules for healthy lifestyle is the feeling of helplessness and hopelessness and people who are depressed or have a low sense of control tend to smoke more, drink more alcohol, eat unhealthily and perform less physical activity. The pathway from stress to disease may therefore follow two lines: one direct via psychobiology, and one indirect via effects on choices of lifestyle (Kristenson *et al.* 2004).

Importantly, these two pathways may have synergistic effects on stress biology: psychological and physical stress work through parallel mechanisms; smoking and alcohol affect cortisol levels, as does food intake of carbohydrates and protein. Therefore, in addition to the behavioural interaction, there may also be a biological interaction where unhealthy lifestyle adds to the burden on the stress system. This synergistic effect between psychosocial factors and lifestyle on psychobiological pathways may be especially important for socio-economic differences in health (Kristenson *et al.* 2004).

Double burden

Social inequalities in health may be a result of double burden; low-status people tend to have more negative exposure and less protective resources. Psychological factors may develop over time in a vicious circle. This leads to a decline from health to ill health; i.e. loss of coping ability leads to strain, to frustration, and, in the next step, to helplessness and hopelessness. These states have both biological and behavioural consequences. The biological stress reactions may develop from a healthy dynamic response to a state of sustained arousal and loss of capacity to respond. The behavioural response may develop from a healthy acceptance of challenge to a depressed loss of initiative and drive for a better life. The direct psychobiological effects of sustained activation and the change in behaviour and motivation form a vicious circle. Repeated negative experience of stressful situations and the use of an unhealthy lifestyle interact and may lead to cumulative effects (Kristenson *et al.* 2004).

Social engineering and paternalism

There is often a debate as to whether to focus on individual responsibility for behaviour (lifestyle and psychosocial factors) or on structural factors. Looking at causes for socio-economic differences in health, it is obvious that structural factors must be the main targets. Reduction of societal polarization, reduction of material deprivation and psychosocial demands and increasing the capacity for support from the social environment will enhance positive outcome expectancies and health. This is also what is aimed at in international, national and regional targets for health, and is the basis for the Ottawa manifest with its focus on health-oriented policies and 'arena perspectives' (Kristenson *et al.* 2004).

However, if focusing only on structural factors, these initiatives may risk becoming 'social engineering' i.e. society created by 'experts' without involvement from people.

The term 'paternalism' is used in debates on ethics. It refers to the 'pater'; the father who does want to do everything he can for his beloved children. However, he is convinced that he, himself, knows best and better than the children what is best for them, and therefore makes his decisions without asking them. All interventions, not least public health interventions and policy decisions in general, have a risk of becoming paternalistic.

The possibilities to intervene on psychological factors

Few programmes for public health include psychological factors as their target. The arguments are that this is not possible to do, and that ambitions to do so would put another burden on people already victimized. But we need to intervene, also, on individual psychosocial factors, i.e. on psychological resources. According to what we have learnt, it is not only the exposure which is important; it is also the ability to handle exposures, the interaction between environment and individual. Power in life is not only a structural factor. It has to be developed by giving people possibilities to take action, to learn, to experience success, to see life as challenges. This can be done (see below) and could also be a way to prevent the paternalistic side-effects of structural interventions.

Empowerment strategies to increase coping ability

The term empowerment is sometimes seen as political dogma. However, it builds on the ambition to enhance individual chances of developing positive expectancies, hopes, self-esteem and trust. A number of studies have shown positive effects of intervention programmes based on empowerment in various study populations, such as people who are chronically ill, individuals suffering from severe pain, patients with cancer and programmes geared at the prevention of HIV in youth (Kristenson *et al.* 2004).

It is important to mention that these positive effects cover clinical parameters as well as psychosocial variables, e.g. depression and quality of life. Empowerment aims at enhancing the potential of people to gain control and to take self-determined actions. Results from a German project, Tackling

Inequalities in Health, indicate that programmes aimed at behavioural change generated positive side-effects. Particularly, those participants who were actively involved in the planning and implementation of the project reported an increase in social integration, self-help and assertiveness (Siegrist and Joksimovic 2001).

Thus, it appears obvious that health promotion interventions should make use of empowerment strategies, since during the process people will gain new learning experiences and will be enabled to meet challenges, to learn new contingencies and to create new, more positive, experiences. In addition to the obvious gain of subjective well-being this may also lead to higher 'toughness' with positive effects on immune function and somatic health development (Dienstbier 1989). This is also an important way to develop supportive societies – since they result from the individuals who build them.

Societal change and health, beyond coping and control

A main argument in this text has been that personal psychosocial resources and coping ability are good for health. While there is rich evidence for this statement, it is still important to be careful about the connotation: coping, in terms of having control, is good as long as there are opportunities for control. Therefore interventions aimed at increasing coping ability must be combined with interventions at structural levels, to create these opportunities. If that is not the case *a need of* control may be deleterious (Siegrist *et al.*1997, Mulatu and Schooler 2002). This has been demonstrated in times of large societal changes e.g. in Sweden during the period 1880–1900 when society changed towards industrialism and urbanism and in Eastern Europe during the decades of transition 1980–2000. The parallels between these developments (one hundred years apart) are striking. A common factor is the dramatic changes in life circumstances which affect people's ability to control their life. A health paradox is seen in both settings with people traditionally regarded as strong i.e. dominant groups (middle-aged men) being most vulnerable to disease and death.

We are today, all over the world, facing rapidly changing societies. This may lead to new health disparities, and even reduced socio-economic differences in health, due to the worsening health for people with high SES. This also puts new demands on stress research. Just as constructs and measures on social and work environments have been developed over the years, so must constructs and measures on personal psychosocial resources and coping be developed. Several of these factors are moderately intercorrelated, and a research strategy that explores their coherence of psychosocial profile that promotes resilience to stress merits empirical examination (Taylor and Seeman 1999). In this research differences between women and men need to be explored more vigorously.

Acknowledgments

This book chapter is, to a large extent, built on the work supported by the European Science Foundation Scientific Programme on Social Variations in Health Expectancy in Europe and special thanks are given to Holger Ursin and Hege Eriksen, of Bergen University, Norway, for collaboration, inspiration and learning on this issue. Also, thanks are given to Judith Sluiter, University of Amsterdam, The Netherlands, and Dagmar Starke University of Düsseldorf, Germany, for the collaboration in former publications which has inspired much of the work in this chapter. For empirical data from the LinQuest study I thank my colleagues in the LinQuest psychobiology group: Elaine Sjögren, Per Leanderson and Jan Ernerudh, Linköping University, Sweden. Finally, thanks are given to Anna Hertting, University of Örebro, Sweden, for constructive criticism of this paper.

References

Adam EK and Gunnar MR (2001). Relationship functioning and home work demands predict individual differences in diurnal cortisol patterns in women. *Psychoneuroendocrinology*, **26**, 189–208.

Adler NE, Epel ES, Castellazzo G and Ickovics R (2000). Relationships of subjective and objective social status with psychological and physiological functioning: preliminary data in healthy white women. *Health Psychology*, **19**, 586–92.

Antonovsky A (1979). *Health, stress and coping: new perspectives on mental and physical well-being*. Jossey Bass, San Francisco.

Brandstädter J, Baltes-Götz B, Kirschbaum C and Hellhammer D (1991). Developmental and personality correlates of adrenocortical activity as indexed by salivary cortisol: observations in the age range of 35–65 years. *Journal of Psychosomatic Research*, **35**, 173–85.

Brydon L, Edwards S, Mohamed-Ali V and Steptoe A (2004). Socio-economic status and stress-induced increases in interleukin-6. *Brain, Behaviour and Immunity*, **18**, 281–90.

Carlsson LE, Speca M, Patel KD and Goodey E (2004). Mindfullness-based stress reduction in relation to quality of life, mood, symptoms of stress and levels of cortisol, dehydroepiandrosterone sulphate (DHEAS) and melantoin in breast and prostata cancer out-patients. *Psychoneuroendocrinology*, **29**, 448–74.

Cohen S, Kaplan GA and Salonen JT (1999). The role of psychological characteristics in the relation between socio-economic status and perceived health. *Journal of Applied Social Psychology*, **29**, 445–68.

Dedert EA, Studts JL, Weissbecker I, Salmon PG, Banis PL and Sephton SE (2004). Religiosity may help preserve the cortisol rhythm in women with stress-related illness. *International Journal of Psychiatry in Medicine*, **34**, 61–77.

Dienstbier R (1989). Arousal and physiological thoughness: implications for mental and physical health. *Psychological Review*, **96**, 84–100.

Hellhammer DH, Buchtal J, Gutberlet I and Kirschbaum C (1997). Social hierarchy and adrenocortical stress reactivity in men. *Psychoneuroendocrinology*, **22**, 643–50.

Hertting A and Theorell T (2002). Physiological changes associated with downsizing of personnel and reorganisation in the health care sector. *Psychotherapy and Psychosomatics*, **71**, 117–22.

Idler EBY (1997). Self-rated health and mortality, a review of twenty-seven community studies. *Journal of Health and Social Behaviour*, **38**, 21–37.

Karasek RA and Theorell T (1990). *Healthy work; stress, productivity and the reconstruction of working life*. Basic Books, New York.

Kiecolt-Glaser JK, McGuire L, Robles TR and Glaser R (2002). Emotions, morbidity and mortality: new perspectives from psychoneuroimmunology. *Annual Review of Psychology*, **53**, 83–107.

Kristenson M (2004). Psychobiological studies of cortisol and interleukin-6. Does method and medium matter? Proceedings from the FCI-meeting in Düsseldorf, November 11–12, 2004.

Kristenson M, Kucinskiene Z, Bergdahl B, Orth-Gomér K (2001). Risk factors for coronary heart disease in different socio-economic groups of Lithuania and Sweden – the LiVicordia study. *Scandinavian Journal of Public Health*, **29**, 140–50.

Kristenson M, Eriksen H, Sluiter J, Starke D and Ursin H (2004). Psychobiological mechanisms of socio-economic differences in health. *Social Science and Medicine*, **58**, 1511–22.

Lachman ME and Weaver SL (1998). The sense of control as a moderator of social class differences in health and well-being. *Journal of Personality and Social Psychology*, **3**, 763–73.

Lantz PM, Lepowski LM, Williams DR, Mero RP and Chen J (1998). Socio-economic factors, health behaviours and mortality. *Journal of American Medical Association*, **279**, 1703–8.

Lynch JW, Kaplan GA, Cohen RD, Tuomilehto T and Salonen JT (1996). Do cardiovascular risk factors explain the relation between socio-economic status, risk of all-cause mortality, cardiovascular mortality, and acute myocardial infarction? *American Journal of Epidemiology*, **144**, 934–42.

Marazziti D and Canale D (2004). Hormonal changes when falling in love. *Psychoneuroendocrinology*, **29**, 931–6.

Marmot MG, Shipley MJ and Rose G (1984). Inequalities in death-specific explanations of a general pattern? *Lancet*, **5**, 1003–6.

Marmot M and Wilkinson R (1999). *Social determinants of health*. Oxford University Press, Oxford.

McEwen BS (2000). The neurobiology of stress: from serendipity to clinical relevance. *Brain Research*, **886**, 172–89.

Mickelson KD and Kubzansky LD (2003). Social distribution of social support: the mediating role of life events. *American Journal of Community Psychology*, **32**, 265–81.

Munck A, Guyre P, and Holbrook N (1984). Physiological functions of glucocorticoids in stress and their relation to pharmacological actions. *Endocrine Reviews*, **5**, 25–44.

Mulato MS and Schooler C (2002). Causal connections between socio-economic status and health: reciprocal effects and mediating mechanisms. *Journal of Health and Social Behaviour*, **43**, 22–41.

Orpana HM and Lemyre L (2004). Explaining the social gradient in health in Canada: using the national population health survey to examine the role of stress. *International Journal of Behavioral Medicine*, **11**, 143–51.

Pearlin L I and Schooler C (1978). The structure of coping. *Journal of Health and Social Behaviour*, **19**, 2–21.

Penninx B, van Tilburg T, Kriegsman DHW, Deeg DJH, Boeke AJP and van Eijk J (1997). Effects of social support and personal coping resources on mortality in older age: the longitudinal aging study Amsterdam. *American Journal of Epidemiology*, **146**, 510–19.

Sephton SE, Sapolsky RM, Kraemer HC and Spiegel D (2000). Diurnal cortisol rhythm as a predictor of breast cancer survival. *Journal of the National Cancer Institute*, **92**, 994–1000.

Siegrist J and Joksimovic L (2001). *Soziale Ungleichheit und Gesundheit in Europa. Teilbericht Deutschland.* BZgA, Köln.

Siegrist J, Klein D and Voigt K-H (1997). Linking sociological with physiological data: the model of effort-reward imbalance at work. *Acta Physiolgica Scandinavica Supplement*, **640**, 112–16.

Siegrist J (2002). Effort-reward imbalance at work and health. In: P Perrewe and D Ganster (eds) *Research in occupational stress and well being, historical and current perspectives on stress and health*, pp. 261–91. JAI Elsevier, New York.

Sjögren E and Kristenson M (2006). Can gender differences in psychosocial factors be explained by socio-economic status? *Scandinavian Journal of Public Health*, **34**, 59–68.

Sjögren E, Leanderson P and Kristenson M (in press). Diurnal saliva cortisol levels and relations to psychosocial factors in a population sample of middle-aged Swedish men and women. *International Journal of Behaviour Medicine*.

Skinner EA (1996). A guide to constructs of control. *Journal of Personality and Social Psychology*, **71**, 549–70.

Steptoe A, Kunz-Ebrecht S, Owen N et al.(2003). Socio-economic status and stress-related biological responses over the working day. *Psychosomatic Medicine*, **65**, 461–70.

Sterling P and Eyer J (1990). Allostasis: a new paradigm to explain arousal pathology. In: S Fisher and J Reason (eds) *Handbook on life stress, cognition and health*, pp. 629–49.Wiley, Chichester.

Surtees P, Wainwright N, Luben R, Khaw KT and Day N (2003). Sense of Coherence and mortality in men and women in the East Norfolk United Kingdom prospective cohort study. *American Journal of Epidemiology*, **15**, 1202–9.

Taylor SE and Seeman TE (1999). Psychosocial resources and the SES-health relationship. *Annals of New York Academy of Sciences*, **896**, 2110–25.

Theorell, T, Hasselhorn H-M, Vingård E, Andersson B, Group MUSIC Norrtälje Study Group (2000). Interleukin-6 and cortisol in acute musculoskeletal disorders: results from a case-referent study in Sweden. *Stress Medicine*, **16**, 27–35.

Ursin H and Eriksen HR (2004). The cognitive activation theory of stress. *Psychoneuroendocrinology*, **29**, 567–92.

van Jaarsveld CHM, Ranchor AV, Sanderman R, Ormel J and Kempen GIJM (2005). The role of premorbid psychological attributes in short- and long-term adjustment after cardiac disease. A prospective study in the elderly in The Netherlands. *Social Science and Medicine*, **60**, 1035–45.

van Lenthe FJ, Schrijvers CTM, Droomers M, Joung IMA, Louwman MI and Mackenbach JP (2004). Investigating explanations for socio-economic inequalities in health. *European Journal of Public Health*, **14**, 63–70.

Chapter 7

Socio-economic differences in health

Are control beliefs fundamental mediators?

Hans Bosma

Introduction

This chapter addresses the role of control beliefs in socio-economic differences in health and provides support for the assumption that low control beliefs might be fundamental mediators in the association between low socio-economic status and poor health. It begins with a socio-historical background to the unhealthy psychological profile in lower socio-economic status groups. The next section presents evidence for low control beliefs being, at least partially, rooted in both childhood and adulthood socio-economic circumstances and the possibility that these beliefs might also be related to the wider socio-economic environment, as defined by neighbourhoods and countries. We then present evidence for low control beliefs being related to heightened risks of disease through varying pathways. Higher depression and hostility levels, as well as adverse health behaviours and a disturbed immune system, may be implicated in these pathways. The contribution of low control beliefs to the socio-economic status–disease association will be quantified in the next section. The possibility that control beliefs may be involved in status attainment processes and the consequences of this for a potential influence of indirect selection are then discussed. Other remaining questions, such as conceptual and empirical issues regarding the control concept, are addressed in the penultimate section. Finally, implications for, and difficulties of, efficient and effective interventions are discussed.

Stigmatization and low control beliefs

Several socio-historical processes in western countries have profoundly pervaded our way of thinking and have resulted in stigmatization of people at the bottom of the socio-economic hierarchy (De Botton 2004). Material conditions and wealth have increased substantially during the twentieth century. Simultaneously, the opportunities to end up in a higher social bracket than one's father or mother have increased. Both processes have strongly elevated expectations which cannot come true for everyone. Rather than accepting low status as a fate or a fait accompli as in pre-modern societies, increasingly low status is associated with feelings of not having attained what could have been attained and with feelings of failure and frustration. Perhaps even more important is the rise of meritocracy (De Botton 2004). 'Meritocracy' refers to the principle that one's social position (the merit) is determined by intelligence and efforts rather than by background characteristics of social origin. The meritocratic principle seems fair and just to many. One drawback, however, is that being at the bottom of the social ranking system in a fully meritocratic society implies that one's intelligence and efforts are considered poor and that one should therefore be blamed for this. While legitimating the socio-economic stratification, the meritocratic principle causes disrespect towards those who are located at the bottom. It is not surprising that feelings of shame, anger, depression, and low self-esteem may arise in these groups. Hence, being poor and deprived is not only intrinsically unpleasant, but is critically reinforced by external pressures that manifest themselves in terms of subtle, but recurrent stigmatization. Thus, the psychological profile of people in lower social classes may be compromised in a systematic way. Several authors have addressed 'low control beliefs' as a major mediator of the association of low socio-economic status with poor health. For instance, Syme discussed the possibility that control beliefs may act as an overarching pathway linking inequalities in societies with health (Syme 1989). According to Syme control beliefs follow a social gradient similar to the inverse social gradient of health that has been documented in many studies (Adler *et al.* 1994, Marmot 2004, Haidt and Rodin 1999). Importantly, low control is associated with poor health and, in addition, low control may be the critical component within diverse explanatory constructs of psychosocial stress, such as low social support or stressful life events. This chapter will elaborate further on the socio-economic roots of low control beliefs and the adverse (health) outcomes that result from these beliefs.

The socio-economic roots of low control beliefs

Emphasizing the socio-economic roots of control beliefs, Wheaton used the terminology 'socialised fatalism' for low control beliefs (Wheaton 1980). Put simply, he stated that 'low socio-economic status in childhood or adult life will socialise individuals to be more fatalistic in their causal perceptions (i.e. to emphasise environmental rather than personal causation of behaviour).

[Socialized fatalism] undermines persistence and effort in coping situations' (Wheaton 1980, p. 101). Using different terminology, but also emphasizing the socio-economic origins of low control beliefs, Ross and Mirowsky (1989) wrote that the 'sense of powerlessness arises from the inability to achieve one's ends, from inadequate resources and opportunities, from restricted alternatives, and from jobs in which one does not choose what to do or how to do it' (Ross and Mirowsky 1989, p. 207). They also agree that 'conditions of powerlessness, structural inconsistency, dependency, and alienated labor are experienced disproportionately by those with low education and low income' (p. 207). The work of Kohn and Schooler is important here. These authors showed that American men in jobs with close supervision, low complexity, and high routinization reported the highest degree of powerlessness, normlessness, and self-estrangement (Kohn and Schooler 1983). Such low control jobs (or jobs with low occupational self-direction) are more common in lower social classes (Bosma et al. 1997, Marmot et al. 1997). In the British Whitehall II study, participants who reported low job control were more likely to be externals, that is, participants who attributed the causes of events (e.g. getting a heart disease) to forces outside themselves. In other words, low job control may generalize to non-work domains (Bosma et al. 1998).

Other research points to the socio-economic determinants of low control beliefs. Findings in the Dutch GLOBE study show that persons whose fathers had a low socio-economic status have lower control beliefs in adulthood and less often use active problem-focused coping than their better-off counterparts (Bosma et al. 1999b). Other psychological factors were similarly, but less strongly, related to background socio-economic status. In this study, reported effects were independent of the adults' own socio-economic status (Figure 7.1). These findings indicate that low control beliefs are partially rooted in childhood social class. As styles of socialization differ among social classes, long-term effects on behaviour, emotion, and cognition may persist into adulthood (Wang et al. 1999). Children from high social class backgrounds may more easily experience a sense of mastery and control because

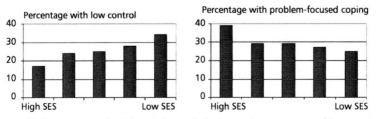

Figure 7.1 Socio-economic status during upbringing and percentages of low control beliefs and active problem-focused coping in adulthood.

their parents have more respective resources. In the same GLOBE study, it was found that adults with a low socio-economic status had an accelerated decrease in control beliefs during the six-year follow-up compared with adults with a high socio-economic status (Bosma *et al.* 1999a). Both GLOBE findings suggest that socio-economic conditions during both upbringing and adulthood impinge on beliefs of control.

The wider socio-economic environment (in adulthood) may also be important. For example, in the Dutch GLOBE study mentioned, it was found that, independent of one's own educational level, persons living in a relatively deprived neighbourhood had higher rates of mortality during the six-year follow-up (Bosma *et al.* 2001). More importantly, in addition to material conditions (poor housing), psychological factors (low control beliefs and passive coping strategies) contributed to this association (Figure 7.2).

Control beliefs may even be important in explaining health differences between countries, as discussed by Marmot and Bobak (2000). These authors specifically point to the importance of control beliefs for explaining differences in life expectancy between Western and Central/Eastern European countries. This line of reasoning is supported by earlier findings from a study of mortality differences between Rotterdam (in the Netherlands) and Kaunas (in Lithuania). In this study, we found that a higher prevalence of poor self-rated health explained the elevated mortality risks in Kaunas substantially, even after controlling for main biological risk factors (Bosma and Appels 1996). In the same Kaunas-Rotterdam Intervention Study (KRIS), it had previously been concluded that a weak sense of mastery may explain the association between poor self-rated health and mortality (Appels *et al.* 1996). These findings support the notion that low control beliefs have their roots at least partially in adverse socio-economic conditions in both childhood and adulthood, and that the wider socio-economic or sociocultural environment may also contribute.

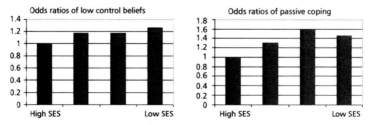

Figure 7.2 Socioeconomic status of the neighbourhood and odds ratios of low control beliefs and passive coping (relative risks).*

* Living in a high SES neighbourhood forms the reference category.

Adverse health outcomes of low control beliefs

Several pathways may operate simultaneously to account for the increased health burden produced by low control beliefs. In this section, three pathways are discussed: (1) a psychological, (2) a behavioural, and (3) a biological pathway. First, let us consider a possible psychological pathway which was described by Melvin Kohn

> An orientational system predicated on conforming to the dictates of authority sees social reality too simply and fearfully to permit taking advantage of options that might otherwise be open. It is too inflexible for precisely those problematic and stressful circumstances that most require subtlety, flexibility, and a perceptive understanding of larger social complexities... [This] suggests that the constricted conditions of life experiences by people of lower social class position foster conceptions of social reality so limited and so rigid as to impair people's ability to deal resourcefully with the problematic and the stressful.
>
> (Kohn 1972, cited in Wheaton 1980, p. 103)

One consequence of this restricted psychological repertoire concerns ineffective modes of coping with adversity. In this view, Wheaton posits that 'socialized fatalism' predisposes low status people to elevated risks of depression as a consequence of failed coping efforts. Similarly, Skinner (1996) points to ineffective and thus, perhaps, unhealthy coping styles of people with low control beliefs. Several studies demonstrated a direct association of low control beliefs with elevated risks of depression in lower socio-economic status groups (Ross and Mirowsky 1989, Haidt and Rodin 1999).

Passive coping in terms of helplessness and depression is one strategy associated with low socio-economic position. Another strategy concerns active coping in terms of anger, aggression, or hostility (Schrijvers *et al.* 2002, Wilkinson 1999). Although hostility in a sense is akin to depressive symptoms, because it taps a negative social attitude, i.e. feelings that others are generally non-supportive and untrustworthy (Scheier and Bridges 1995), anger and aggression tap a more outward-directed active expression of poor mental well-being. The extent to which a continuous struggle with chronic stress in the form of low control-induced maladaptive coping results in vital exhaustion or chronic fatigue needs further examination, but seems not unlikely (Appels *et al.* 1997).

In summary, maladaptive coping as evidenced by helplessness and depression (more passive response to low control), hostility and anger (more active response to low control), or vital exhaustion seems to be associated with low control beliefs. As all these conditions are more prevalent among lower socio-economic groups, the question arises as to how this might mediate the association between low status and disease. In general, two pathways are considered: adverse health behaviours and excessive psychobiological stress reactions.

The pathway through health behaviours, such as smoking, exercise, and alcohol consumption, may be important. This is exemplified by the relevant position of self-efficacy in models of behavioural change (e.g. Ajzen, 1991, Leganger and Kraft 2003). These studies indicate that persons with low control beliefs more frequently think that they cannot quit smoking (or cannot avoid starting to smoke), cannot increase leisure-time physical exercise, and cannot decrease their consumption of alcoholic beverages. It is also possible that they more frequently think that these behaviours do not matter for their health. Given the resulting higher probability of adverse health behaviours in these individuals, it comes as no surprise that risks of disease are likely to be elevated.

There is comparable evidence that stress-induced neuroendocrine or immunological pathways are implicated (Haidt and Rodin 1999, Krantz and McCeney 2002, Kristenson *et al.* 2004, McEwen and Seeman 1999, Skinner 1996; see also Chapters 5 and 6 in this volume). The initially healthy biological responses to stressors are increasingly compromised when stressors become chronic, and these conditions are more frequent in lower socio-economic status groups (Kristenson *et al.* 2004). The continuous biological wear and tear leads to an elevated allostatic load in low socio-economic status groups where there is 'no margin left for responding to additional challenges and no opportunities for relaxation' (Kristenson *et al.* 2004, p. 1515). In their review, Kristenson and colleagues conclude: 'The direct pathophysiological effects of SES and sustained activation relate to metabolic disturbances such as insulin resistance, tissue damage in inflammation, infections and immunology, fluid loss, neurochemical activity and oxidative stress reactions' (Kristenson *et al.* 2004, p. 1515). Other studies generally confirm the adverse influence of uncontrollability or the belief therein on cardiovascular, endocrine, and immune function (e.g. Chen *et al.* 2003, Kunz-Ebrecht *et al.* 2004).

Some quantifications

Empirical evidence supporting the socio-economic status–control beliefs–health pathway is illustrated in Figure 7.3. On the left, the figure presents findings from the Dutch longitudinal GLOBE study regarding the influence of low socio-economic status during upbringing on self-rated poor health in adulthood. When adjusting for the variable 'control beliefs' it becomes apparent that about a third to one half of this association is accounted for by a higher prevalence of low control beliefs in the adults that grew up in adverse socio-economic conditions (Bosma *et al.* 1999b). On the right side, Figure 7.3 presents the influence of low control beliefs on the association between

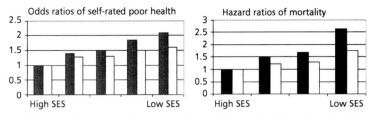

Figure 7.3 Low socio-economic status during upbringing (left figure) and adulthood (right figure) and risks of self-rated poor health and mortality, respectively, before (black bar) and after (white bar) control for low control beliefs (relative risks).*

* High SES forms the reference category.

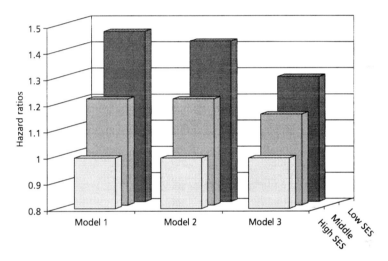

Figure 7.4 Socio-economic status and hazard ratios of heart disease, controlled for age and sex (model 1), additionally controlled for health behaviours (model 2), and additionally controlled for control beliefs (model 3) (relative risks).*

* High SES forms the reference category.

socio-economic status (as measured by education) and mortality during the six-year follow-up. Again, up to half of this association is 'explained' by low control beliefs (Bosma *et al.* 1999a).

Another recent Dutch study (GLAS) confirmed that the contribution of control beliefs to the association between socio-economic status and heart disease may be substantial (Bosma *et al.* 2005). In this five-year follow-up study among men and women aged 57 and older, low control beliefs in the lower socio-economic status groups took into account about a third of the socio-economic differences in incident heart disease (Figure 7.4). This figure also shows that the pathway via control beliefs is largely independent of the pathway through health behaviours and other classical coronary risk factors. This suggests an important pathway via physiological mechanisms (see the previous section).

The possibility of indirect selection via control beliefs

Observing socio-demographic variations in control beliefs, Lachman and Weaver concluded that – given the cross-sectional design of their study

> It is not possible to determine whether education leads to a greater sense of control because of more opportunities and resources or whether those who have a greater sense of control were the ones more likely to seek advanced education. Those who have higher control beliefs should be more motivated to pursue higher education because they believe they are able to bring about desired outcomes and education is one means to facilitate this.
>
> (Lachman and Weaver 1998a, p. 560)

More direct evidence on the importance of control beliefs for status attainment processes is now available. For example, using data from the (US) National Longitudinal Survey of Young Women, Osborne (2000) found that women with low control beliefs have lower incomes than women with high control beliefs. A one standard deviation increase in 'fatalism' was estimated to be related to a decrease of 7 per cent in income. Importantly, this effect was independent of years of schooling, intelligence, work experience, number of children, and socio-economic status of the parents. Wang and colleagues (1999) examined 2,000 American senior high school students in 1972. The students were reassessed in 1979 (age 25) and in 1986 (age 32). These authors found that psychological factors, such as high self-esteem and internal locus of control (i.e. favourable control beliefs), had strong positive effects on educational and occupational attainment. The effect of high control beliefs was independent of – and even stronger than – the effect of parental education or occupation (Figure 7.5).

These studies suggest that control beliefs may act as a critical confounder rather than as a fundamental mediator in the association between socio-economic status and disease risks. Given the evidence that low control increases morbidity and mortality, there is reason to believe that indirect selection may play a role and that the contribution of socio-economic status towards explaining health variations may have been overestimated. Furthermore, we cannot rule out that control beliefs, to some extent, are hereditary, as is the case with several personality characteristics (Johansson et al. 2001). This fact might

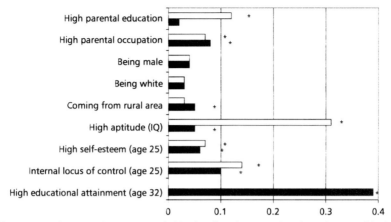

Figure 7.5 Educational attainment (white bars) and occupational attainment (black bars) at age 32 as predicted by family background, demographic characteristics, aptitude, and psychological characteristics (simultaneously controlled; standardised regression coefficients).* Copyright 1999. From status attainment in America: the roles of locus of control and self-esteem in educational and occupational outcomes by Wang LY, Kick E, Fraser J, Burns TJ in *Sociological Spectrum*. Reproduced by permission of Taylor and Francis Group, LLC., http://www.taylor and francis.com.
* $p < 0.05$.

further complicate the analysis of associations under study. The extent to which genetic influences, individual factors, such as control beliefs, and socio-economic circumstances in childhood and adulthood interact in producing differential illness susceptibility remains to be unravelled (Holtzman 2002). What is more important now is the observation that control beliefs are simultaneously involved in status attainment processes and in disease development. Future research will have to estimate the extent of this indirect selection using appropriate longitudinal study designs, preferably birth cohorts. It may well be that socio-economic circumstances and control beliefs work in tandem in a reciprocal relationship during the whole life course.

Other remaining issues

Several issues need further consideration when discussing control beliefs. First, control beliefs are individual perceptions, and further research is needed regarding the extent to which these perceptions are subjective reflections of objective environmental factors that are in or out of control. The question then becomes one of whether adverse effects of low control beliefs are perhaps confounded by environmental factors, such as socio-economic adversity or low control and autonomy at work. This, of course, is of considerable importance for intervention purposes. When low control beliefs are not fully reflective of the objective environment (e.g. if there is variation in control beliefs within separate socio-economic groups), it is important to know whether control beliefs have equally beneficial effects on health in persons in rich and poor (socio-economic) environments. Questions such as the following remain unanswered today: Do control beliefs have similarly beneficial effects on health in all socio-economic status groups, or is their beneficial effect restricted to low socio-economic status groups (see e.g. Lachman *et al.* 1998b, Landau 1995)? And to what extent are control beliefs beneficial for health even if they do not match with objective control-limiting conditions?

Second, more research is needed on how the different control concepts contribute to the explanation of adverse health (Skinner 1996). For instance, co-manifestation of low self-efficacy (e.g. thinking that one cannot quit smoking) and high mastery (e.g. thinking that quitting protects against heart disease) may particularly aggravate adverse health. Third, more research is also needed regarding how the concept of 'desire for control' combines with self-efficacy and mastery in the prediction of health (Burger 1992). For example, one could assume that low self-efficacy in combination with poor mastery beliefs affects health outcomes particularly strongly in persons who exhibit a high desire for control, whereas effects are less pronounced in other groups. Striving for control when there is little chance of achieving real control is likely to produce strongest effects. On the other hand, a low desire for (internal) control, combined with a high external control belief, as in persons with a strong and satisfying belief in divine power, may be related to beneficial health outcomes. In this context, several studies suggest that control beliefs have an optimal level or threshold above which health benefits decline (e.g. Wheaton 1980). These unresolved issues can help to explain why some researchers did not find evidence for positive effects of control beliefs on health and why the mediation hypothesis of control beliefs in accounting for socio-economic differences in health does not always receive unequivocal support (e.g. Pikhart *et al.* 2003, Schwartz 2000, Seeman 1991).

Possibilities for interventions

To reduce socio-economic differences in health, one might focus upon reducing socio-economic inequality itself, upon reducing the consequences of socio-economic differences, upon reducing the negative effects of health problems on indicators of socio-economic status (direct selection), or upon improving access to and effectiveness of health care for lower socio-economic status groups (Mackenbach and Bakker 2003, see also Chapter 10 in this volume). The research presented in this chapter indicates that low control beliefs are a major consequence of socio-economic status and an important contributor to poor health outcomes. Furthermore, the possibility of indirect selection via control beliefs and the finding that positive control beliefs may be particularly protective for health in low socio-economic status groups (Lachman and Weaver 1998b, Landau 1995), point to the potential usefulness of targeting control beliefs in interventions directed at reducing socio-economic differences in health.

One such strategy concerns the empowerment of people with low control beliefs. For example, hoping for positive changes in the quality of life, experts recommended an increase in self-management skills of people with low self-efficacy (e.g. Lorig and Holman 2003). Given the higher prevalence of low control beliefs (and the potentially stronger adverse effects of these beliefs) in low socio-economic status groups, socio-economic differences in health outcomes can be expected to decrease. These proposed interventions include health care development in addition to skills training programmes, and these interventions are directed towards both healthy and chronically ill people. Yet we need to have better knowledge on how health care services can be modified to promote control beliefs in both primary and secondary prevention efforts.

Keeping in mind our previous arguments, it is of utmost importance to intervene at the structural level as well, because structural constraints are powerful determinants of low control beliefs. Otherwise, there is a risk of 'blaming the victim' instead of inducing real change (Muntaner 2004, Muntaner and Lynch 1999). Some proponents have therefore developed an ecological approach towards empowerment. This means that communities (neighbourhoods) should be empowered, e.g. by increasing the social networks within the neighbourhood (Wallerstein 2002). This will increase collective efficacy (Haidt and Rodin 1999). As Syme again noted: 'While control is a characteristic of individuals, it is also a product of the environment' (Syme 1989, p. 11). Control beliefs are rooted, shaped and maintained in environments with control-limiting obstacles or values. Therefore, interventions should be directed at both the environment and the individuals. Probably most effective is an approach in which attempts are made to increase control beliefs in combination with increases in actual power. The latter is brought about by decreasing income inequalities, avoiding absolute deprivation, and improving physical and psychosocial working, housing, and neighbourhood conditions (Mackenbach and Bakker 2003). Inter-sectoral policies at governmental level are needed to tackle socio-economic differences in health in an efficient way.

In conclusion, control beliefs are an important mediator in socio-economic differences in health. We have argued that low control beliefs may underlie socio-economic differences in health between and within countries. Deprivation and material factors are also important, but their influence probably is restricted to the lower end of the socio-economic hierarchy, and these factors partly affect health through control beliefs. The current conclusion that control beliefs might be a fundamental mediator is based on two observations, first that low control beliefs are (partially) rooted in and shaped by adverse socio-economic conditions during upbringing and adulthood, and second that low control beliefs are related to adverse health outcomes through complex psychological, behavioural, and biological pathways. The possibility of indirect selection via control beliefs and the dilemma of structural versus individual interventions need further elaboration.

Acknowledgements

Here I would like to thank the European Science Foundation (ESF) Scientific Programme on Social Variations in Health Expectancy in Europe and its members for their support and inspiration. I am particularly grateful to (in alphabetical order) Ad Appels, Jan De Jonge, Ruud Kempen, Johan Mackenbach, Michael Marmot, Johannes Siegrist, Jacques Van Eijck, and Frank Van Lenthe and their teams for use of their data and inspiring thoughts.

References

Adler NE, Boyce T, Chesney MA *et al.* (1994). Socioeconomic status and health. The challenge of the gradient. *American Psychologist*, **49**, 15–24.

Ajzen I (1991). The theory of planned behavior. *Organizational Behavior and Human Decision Processes*, **50**, 179–211.

Appels A, Siegrist J, De Vos Y (1997). Chronic workload, need for control and vital exhaustion in patients with myocardial infarction and controls: a comparative test of cardiovascular risk profiles. *Stress Medicine*, **13**, 117–21.

Appels A, Bosma H, Grabauskas V, Gostautas A, Sturmans F (1996). Self-rated health and mortality in a Lithuanian and a Dutch population. *Social Science and Medicine*, **42**, 681–9.

Bosma H and Appels A (1996). Differences in mortality between Lithuanian and Dutch middle-aged men. Results from the Kaunas-Rotterdam Intervention Study. In: C Hertzman, S Kelly, M Bobak (eds) *East-west life expectancy gap in Europe. Environmental and non-environmental determinants*, pp. 161–7. Kluwer Academic Publishers, Amsterdam.

Bosma H, Schrijvers C, Mackenbach JP (1999a). Socioeconomic inequalities in mortality and importance of perceived control: cohort study. *British Medical Journal*, **319**, 1469–70.

Bosma H, Stansfeld SA, Marmot MG (1998). Job control, personal characteristics, and heart disease. *Journal of Occupational Health Psychology*, **3**, 402–9.

Bosma H, van de Mheen HD, Mackenbach JP (1999b). Social class in childhood and general health in adulthood: questionnaire study of contribution of psychological attributes. *British Medical Journal*, **318**, 18–22.

Bosma H, van de Mheen HD, Borsboom GJ, Mackenbach JP (2001). Neighborhood socio-economic status and all-cause mortality. *American Journal of Epidemiology*, **153**, 363–71.

Bosma H, Marmot MG, Hemingway H, Nicholson AC, Brunner E, Stansfeld SA (1997). Low job control and risk of coronary heart disease in Whitehall II (prospective cohort) study. *British Medical Journal*, **314**, 558–65.

Bosma H, Van Jaarsveld CHM, Tuinstra J *et al.* (2005). Low control beliefs, classical coronary risk factors, and socio-economic differences in heart disease in older persons. *Social Science and Medicine*, **60**, 737–45.

Burger JM (1992). *Desire for control: personality, social and clinical perspectives*. Plenum, New York.

Chen E, Fisher EB, Bacharier LB, Strunk RC (2003). Socioeconomic status, stress, and immune markers in adolescents with asthma. *Psychosomatic Medicine*, **65**, 984–92.

De Botton A (2004). *Status anxiety*. Hamish Hamilton, London.

Haidt J and Rodin J (1999). Control and efficacy as interdisciplinary bridges. *Review of General Psychology*, **3**, 317–37.

Holtzman NA (2002). Genetics and social class. *Journal of Epidemiology and Community Health*, **56**, 529–35.

Johansson B, Grant JD, Plomin R *et al.* (2001). Health locus of control in late life: a study of genetic and environmental influences in twins aged 80 years and older. *Health Psychology*, **20**, 33–40.

Kohn ML (1972). Class, family, and schizophrenia. *Social Forces*, **50**, 295–302.

Kohn ML and Schooler C (1983). *Work and personality: an inquiry into the impact of social stratification*. Ablex, Norwood, NJ.

Krantz DS and McCeney MK (2002). Effects of psychological and social factors on organic disease: a critical assessment of research on coronary heart disease. *Annual Review of Psychology*, **53**, 341–69.

Kristenson M, Eriksen HR, Sluiter JK, Starke D, Ursin H (2004). Psychobiological mechanisms of socio-economic differences in health. *Social Science and Medicine*, **58**, 1511–22.

Kunz-Ebrecht SR, Kirschbaum C, Marmot M, Steptoe A (2004). Differences in cortisol awakening response on work days and weekends in women and men from the Whitehall II cohort. *Psychoneuroendocrinology*, **29**, 516–28.

Lachman ME and Weaver SL (1998a). Sociodemographic variations in the sense of control by domain: findings from the MacArthur studies of midlife. *Psychology and Aging*, **13**, 553–62.

Lachman ME and Weaver SL (1998b). The sense of control as a moderator of social class differences in health and well-being. *Journal of Personality and Social Psychology*, **74**, 763–73.

Landau R (1995). Locus of control and socio-economic status: does internal locus of control reflect real resources and opportunities or personal coping abilities? *Social Science and Medicine*, **41**, 1499–505.

Leganger A and Kraft P (2003). Control constructs: do they mediate the relation between educational attainment and health behaviour? *Journal of Health Psychology*, **8**, 361–72.

Lorig KR and Holman H (2003). Self-management education: history, definition, outcomes, and mechanisms. *Annals of Behavorial Medicine*, **26**, 1–7.

Mackenbach JP and Bakker MJ, European Network on Interventions and Policies to Reduce Inequalities in Health (2003). Tackling socio-economic inequalities in health: analysis of European experiences. *Lancet*, **362**, 1409–14.

Marmot M (2004). *Status syndrome. How our position on the social gradient affects longevity and health.* Bloomsbury Publishing, London.

Marmot M and Bobak M (2000). International comparators and poverty and health in Europe. *British Medical Journal*, **321**, 1124–8.

Marmot MG, Bosma H, Hemingway H, Brunner E, Stansfeld S (1997). Contribution of job control and other risk factors to social variations in coronary heart disease incidence. *Lancet*, **350**, 235–9.

McEwen BS and Seeman T (1999). Protective and damaging effects of mediators of stress. Elaborating and testing the concepts of allostasis and allostatic load. *Annals of the New York Academy of Sciences*, **896**, 30–47.

Muntaner C (2004). Commentary: Social capital, social class, and the slow progress of psychosocial epidemiology. *International Journal of Epidemiology*, **33**, 674–80.

Muntaner C and Lynch J (1999). Income inequality, social cohesion, and class relations: a critique of Wilkinson's neo-Durkheimian research program. *International Journal of Health Services*, **29**, 59–81.

Osborne M (2000). *The power of personality: labor market rewards and the transmission of earnings.* University of Massachusetts, Massachusetts.

Pikhart H, Bobak M, Rose R, Marmot M (2003). Household item ownership and self-rated health: material and psychosocial explanations. *BMC Public Health*, **3**, 38.

Ross CE and Mirowsky J (1989). Explaining the social patterns of depression: control and problem solving – or support and talking? *Journal of Health and Social Behavior*, **30**, 206–19.

Scheier MF and Bridges MW (1995). Person variables and health: personality predispositions and acute psychological states as shared determinants for disease. *Psychosomatic Medicine*, **57**, 255–68.

Schrijvers CT, Bosma H, Mackenbach JP (2002). Hostility and the educational gradient in health. The mediating role of health-related behaviours. *European Journal of Public Health*, **12**, 110–16.

Schwartz B (2000). Self-determination. The tyranny of freedom. *American Psychologist*, **55**, 79–88.

Seeman M (1991). Alienation and anomie. In: JP Robinson, PR Shaver, LS Wrightsman (eds) *Measures of personality and social psychological attitudes*, vol. 1, pp. 291–372. Academic Press Inc., San Diego, CA.

Skinner EA (1996). A guide to constructs of control. *Journal of Personality and Social Psychology*, **71**, 549–70.

Syme SL (1989). Control and health: a personal perspective. In: A Steptoe and A Appels (eds) *Stress, personal control and health*, pp. 3–18. Wiley, London.

Wallerstein N (2002). Empowerment to reduce health disparities. *Scandinavian Journal of Public Health*, Suppl., **59**, 72–7.

Wang LY, Kick E, Fraser J, Burns TJ (1999). Status attainment in America: the roles of locus of control and self-esteem in educational and occupational outcomes. *Sociological Spectrum*, **19**, 281–98.

Wheaton B (1980). The sociogenesis of psychological disorder: an attributional theory. *Journal of Health and Social Behavior*, **21**, 100–24.

Wilkinson RG (1999). Health, hierarchy, and social anxiety. *Annals of the New York Academy of Sciences*, **896**, 48–63.

Chapter 8

Aggregate deprivation and effects on health

Frank J. van Lenthe

Introduction

Empirical evidence showing that mortality rates for neighbourhoods are patterned by neighbourhood poverty and wealth had already been reported in the early nineteenth century (Villermé 1826). Theoretically, these findings could be explained by the composition of the neighbourhoods with regard to age, sex or individual-level socio-economic position of the residents; poor neighbourhoods mainly host poor people with an increased risk of mortality. Alternatively, these higher mortality rates in the poverty areas could also be due to neighbourhood characteristics to which all neighbourhood residents were exposed, such as the availability and quality of water. The question of whether living in more deprived neighbourhoods was related to poorer health because of the socio-economic characteristics of neighbourhood residents (often called a 'compositional' effect) or due to characteristics of the neigh-bourhood (often called a 'contextual' effect) remained unsolved for a long time: individual-level socio-economic data were hardly available in these early studies, and associations found at the neighbourhood level could not be translated to the individual level.

The publication of the Black Report in England in 1980 (Townsend and Davidson 1982), demonstrating socio-economic inequalities in health in the United Kingdom, revitalized research on socio-economic inequalities in health in many Western societies. Prospective studies showed an inverse asso-ciation between socio-economic position and health; often these differences could not be fully explained by the higher prevalence of well-known biological or behavioural risk factors of major chronic diseases (Marmot *et al.* 1991). The extent to which these inequalities were driven by area-level characteristics was unclear. Methodological improvements nowadays allow the inclusion of variables at different levels in statistical analyses. Recent studies have used multi-level analyses to examine whether associations of neighbourhood socio-economic environment with mortality are the result of a compositional effect.

In an early example from the US, Haan *et al.* (1987) showed an increased risk of death for residents living in poverty areas. In order to test whether this association was due to the composition of residents in terms of their individual-level socio-economic position, the analyses were additionally adjusted for individual-level socio-economic factors. The increased risk of mortality of living in the poverty areas reduced, indicating that part of the increased risk was indeed due to the higher prevalence of participants with a low socio-economic position in the poverty areas. However, significantly increased mortality risks remained after the adjustment, indicating that contextual factors could contribute to the increased risk as well. Several, though not all (Slogett and Joshi 1994, Veugelers *et al.* 2001) subsequent studies reported essentially similar findings (Picket and Pearl 2001, Bosma *et al.* 2001, Martikainen *et al.* 2003, Borell *et al.* 2004, Marinacci *et al.* 2004). Thus, there seems to be an increased risk of premature mortality of living in more deprived neighbourhoods, regardless of individual-level education, occupation or income. Similar increased risk has also been found for chronic diseases such as coronary heart diseases, and their classical biological and behavioural risk factors (Picket and Pearl 2001).

These findings have important implications. First, characteristics of the place of residence determine health, and these characteristics may generally be more unfavourable for those in the lower socio-economic groups compared to those in higher socio-economic groups. As such, neighbourhood characteristics may contribute to the explanation of socio-economic inequalities in health. Second, given the clustering of good and poor health by the neighbourhood socio-economic environment, the neighbourhood may serve as a setting for interventions. These interventions may aim to change both individual and neighbourhood characteristics. Given that the majority of residents in more deprived neighbourhoods are from lower socio-economic groups, such interventions could contribute to the actual reduction of the health gap between those from lower and higher socio-economic groups. However, the advancement of understanding socio-economic inequalities in health through the inclusion of neighbourhood characteristics, and using the neighbourhood as a setting for interventions, requires that the processes underlying the association between the neighbourhood socio-economic environment and health is much better understood.

The purpose of this chapter is to contribute to the improvement of this understanding through an international comparison of the size of the association between the neighbourhood socio-economic environment and health. In addition, an overview of some important conceptual and methodological issues, which need to be solved for the advancement of this understanding, will be described. Finally, policy implications of the results will be outlined.

Explaining neighbourhood inequalities in health: an international comparison

One approach to improve our understanding about the processes linking the neighbourhood socio-economic environment to health is to compare data across several countries. The presence of differences in these associations across countries would prompt further investigation of what specific country-level factors enhance or attenuate neighbourhood effects. There are several reasons why the size of the association between the neighbourhood socio-economic environment and health may differ between countries. First, the range in absolute levels of the neighbourhood socio-economic environment may differ from country to country. Thus, mortality differences between the lowest and highest levels of the socio-economic environment across countries could result simply from the fact that the ranges compared differ from country to country. Second, there may be differences in residential segregation by socio-economic position between countries. It may be expected that the larger the residential segregation by socio-economic position, the stronger the association between the neighbourhood socio-economic environment and health. The degree of segregation may be the result of national policies, for example social housing policies. As such, country-level policies may contribute to increasing or decreasing neighbourhood effects on health.

Similarly, the provision of welfare and public services may be of higher quality and may be distributed more uniformly in some countries, which may reduce the health impact of living in disadvantaged neighbourhoods. It has been argued, for example, that the stronger association between income inequality and mortality in the US compared to Canada may be explained by the universal availability of publicly funded services in Canada compared with the market-led provision of services in the US (Ross *et al.* 2000). Third, differences in the physical and social environment between advantaged and more disadvantaged neighbourhoods may differ between countries. A fourth possible reason for country-specific effects of the neighbourhood socio-economic environment on mortality is a difference in exposure to the neighbourhood. Differences in rates of residential mobility along with patterns of working and socializing outside the local area could lead to differential exposure across countries.

Until now, comparisons of the association between the neighbourhood socio-economic environment and health between studies have been hampered by methodological differences. Recently, however, associations were compared between public sector employees in London and Helsinki (Stafford *et al.* 2004). The neighbourhood socio-economic environment, as measured for example by the neighbourhood unemployment, was related to self-rated health in both countries and no clear differences in the size of these associations were found between both cities. Using an index of dissimilarity, a higher degree of residential segregation was demonstrated in London compared to Helsinki and this was coupled with some greater variation in self-rated health between neighbourhoods in London compared to Helsinki.

To compare the size of the association between the neighbourhood socio-economic environment and health (i.e. all-cause mortality) over a broader range of countries, data were obtained from three prospective studies in which selected samples were followed over time (the ARIC study in the US, the GLOBE study in the Netherlands, and the Whitehall II study in the UK) (Marmot *et al.* 1991, The ARIC Investigators 1989, Mackenbach *et al.* 1994) and three population-based registry studies in Helsinki (Finland) (Martikainen *et al.* 2003), Turin (Italy) (Cardano *et al.* 2004) and Madrid (Spain) (Regidor *et al.* 2002), based on coverage of almost the entire general population in the areas using death-registry information.

The ARIC study was carried out in four US regions. In three of the four regions, the population reflects the demographic composition of the communities from which they were chosen (with predominantly, but not exclusively, whites). In the fourth region (Jackson) only blacks were sampled. In order to make the six study populations more comparable (and because the investigation of ethnic differences raises additional issues) the analyses in the ARIC study were restricted to the three regions including mainly whites. Neighbourhoods were defined using existing administrative or geographical boundaries with the median number of residents per neighbourhood varying from n = 1,220 in the study in Madrid to n = 14,090 in the study in Helsinki. The mean age of the participants was about 45 years in all studies, with participants in the ARIC and GLOBE study being slightly older on average. All studies included approximately equal numbers of males and females, except in Whitehall II (the majority being males) and Helsinki (only males included).

Neighbourhood unemployment was used as an indicator of the neighbourhood socio-economic environment. Unemployment was selected as the neighbourhood indicator because it was the variable that was available systematically across studies. Information on unemployment rates was derived from census-based data in all studies.

In all countries except Spain and the US, neighbourhood unemployment was calculated by dividing the number of unemployed persons (e.g. actively seeking employment, thus excluding housewives, retirees and students) by the total number of persons in the working age population (in general between 15 and 65 years of age). In Spain and the US, neighbourhood unemployment was defined as the population of unemployed persons among the economically active population in the working age population. Thus, instead of the entire working age population, the denominator in the Spanish and US definitions excluded persons not economically active or not in the labour force (e.g. housewives, students, retirees). The substantial higher neighbourhood unemployment rates in Spain may be partly caused by this methodological deviation from the other studies, but they are also 'real', as Spain is among the European countries with the highest unemployment rates.

Socioeconomic characteristics at the individual-level included education and occupation. Maximum efforts were made to make these variables similar across countries.

Although different approaches were used to collect information on mortality, all studies had nearly complete mortality data, with the exception of the study in Madrid. In the latter study, the population census and the 1996 and 1997 mortality registries could be successfully linked for 70 per cent of the deceased persons, but there were no significant socio-economic or sociodemographic differences between deceased persons linked and not linked. A more detailed description of the methods is presented elsewhere (Van Lenthe *et al.* 2005). Table 8.1 includes descriptive information about the studies included.

Country-specific cut-off points of quartiles of neighbourhood unemployment were approximately similar in the ARIC, GLOBE and Whitehall II studies and in Turin (Table 8.1). Cut-off points of quartiles of neighbourhood unemployment were substantially lower in Helsinki, and substantially higher in Madrid.

Cox proportional hazard models were used to assess the association between neighbourhood unemployment and mortality. The resulting hazard ratios (HR) in Table 8.2 can be interpreted as the relative risks of mortality during the follow-up period in each quartile of neighbourhood unemployment compared with this risk in the quartile of neighbourhoods with the lowest neighbourhood unemployment. In model 1 in Table 8.2, the association was adjusted for individual age of study participants. By adjusting for age, we took into account that the age distribution may vary between neighbourhoods, and that in neighbourhoods with many elderly participants the relative risk of mortality is higher. In model 2, we additionally adjusted for education and occupation of participants. The reduction in the relative risk of mortality by neighbourhood unemployment rates as a consequence of this adjustment can be interpreted as the contribution of individual-level education and occupation to the increased relative risks of living in neighbourhoods with high unemployment rates (a compositional effect). The remaining relative risks after these adjustments can be due to compositional factors for which we did not adjust, or to contextual factors.

Table 8.1 Descriptive information by quartiles of neighbourhood unemployment

	Neighbourhood unemployment (quartiles)			
	1 (least unemployment)	2	3	4 (most unemployment)
Unemployment cut points (%)*				
ARIC	< 1.9	1.9–3.5	3.5–5.4	> 5.4
GLOBE	< 4.8	4.8–7.7	7.8–9.7	> 9.7
Whitehall II	< 3.9	3.9–5.1	5.2–7.6	> 7.6
Helsinki	< 1.02	1.02–1.30	1.31–1.63	> 1.63
Turin	< 6.2	6.2–8.2	8.3–10.2	> 10.2
Madrid	< 18.8	18.8–21.8	21.9–25.3	> 25.3
Low education (%)**				
ARIC	13.3	16.9	19.8	22.8
GLOBE	11.2	24.6	22.6	30.1
Whitehall II	4.7	7.0	7.1	11.5
Helsinki	28.4	33.5	36.3	41.0
Turin	19.8	28.5	33.2	40.2
Madrid	19.1	30.0	40.3	51.6
Higher grade professionals***				
ARIC	32.6	29.1	24.0	20.6
GLOBE	14.2	6.3	6.4	5.5
Whitehall II	42.4	36.7	27.0	16.0
Helsinki	37.3	29.2	25.0	19.8
Turin	4.9	2.0	1.6	0.8
Madrid	39.8	26.7	16.3	8.9

* Quartiles are derived from census-based data.

** Definitions of lowest education: ARIC: less than high school, GLOBE: primary school, Whitehall II: no academic qualifications, Helsinki: up to nine years of education, Turin: primary, Madrid: primary education and lower.

*** Highest categories are presented because they are more comparable between countries than the lowest occupational categories. Definitions are: ARIC: executive, managerial and professional, GLOBE: higher grade professionals, Whitehall II: higher (executives, top managers), Helsinki: upper white collar, Turin: higher grade white collar, Madrid: higher grade professionals.

Source: Van Lenthe et al. (2005). Journal of Epidemiology and Community Health, **59**, 223–30 (reprinted with permission).

Table 8.2 Sex-specific hazard ratios for all cause mortality according to neighbourhood unemployment before and after adjustment for individual socio-economic indicators

	Males		Females	
	Hazard ratio (95% confidence interval)		Hazard ratio (95% confidence interval)	
	Model 1*	Model 2	Model 1*	Model 2
ARIC				
1. (least unemployment)	1.00	1.00	1.00	1.00
2.	1.11 (0.88–1.41)	1.08 (0.85–1.38)	1.41 (0.99–2.01)	1.40 (1.00–1.97)
3.	1.36 (1.08–1.71)	1.29 (1.03–1.61)	1.44 (1.05–1.97)	1.38 (1.01–1.88)
4. (most unemployment)	1.32 (1.04–1.68)	1.21 (0.96–1.53)	1.75 (1.28–2.40)	1.63 (1.20–2.22)
Percentage reduction in hazard ratio**		34%		16%
GLOBE				
1. (least unemployment)	1.00	1.00	1.00	1.00
2.	1.22 (0.97–1.55)	1.12 (0.89–1.41)	1.23 (0.86–1.77)	1.13 (0.80–1.61)
3.	1.22 (0.91–1.54)	1.11 (0.84–1.47)	1.36 (0.91–2.02)	1.26 (0.85–1.87)
4. (most unemployment)	1.67 (1.25–2.22)	1.46 (1.09–1.95)	1.33 (0.83–2.13)	1.19 (0.77–1.85)
Percentage reduction in hazard ratio		31%		42%
Whitehall II				
1. (least unemployment)	1.00	1.00	1.00	1.00
2.	1.17 (0.83–1.65)	1.05 (0.71–1.56)	0.92 (0.46–1.86)	1.10 (0.50–2.43)
3.	1.40 (1.00–1.98)	1.21 (0.83–1.76)	0.77 (0.44–1.50)	0.78 (0.36–1.66)
4. (most unemployment)	1.70 (1.22–2.36)	1.19 (0.79–1.78)	1.39 (0.78–2.46)	1.26 (0.64–2.46)
Percentage reduction in hazard ratio		73%		33%

Table 8.2 (*Continued*)

| | Males | | Females | |
| | Hazard ratio (95% confidence interval) | | Hazard ratio (95% confidence interval) | |
	Model 1*	Model 2	Model 1*	Model 2
Helsinki				
1. (least unemployment)	1.00	1.00		
2.	1.21 (1.08–1.35)	1.14 (1.03–1.25)		
3.	1.34 (1.20–1.50)	1.22 (1.11–1.34)		
4. (most unemployment)	1.67 (1.50–1.86)	1.41 (1.28–1.55)		
Percentage reduction in hazard ratio		39%		
Turin				
1. (least unemployment)	1.00	1.00	1.00	1.00
2.	1.09 (1.03–1.16)	1.02 (0.96–1.09)	1.06 (0.95–1.13)	1.04 (0.97–1.10)
3.	1.20 (1.14–1.27)	1.10 (1.02–1.18)	1.14 (1.07–1.21)	1.11 (1.04–1.18)
4. (most unemployment)	1.28 (1.23–1.35)	1.14 (1.07–1.21)	1.16 (1.09–1.24)	1.12 (1.05–1.20)
Percentage reduction in hazard ratio		50%		25%
Madrid				
1. Least unemployment	1.00	1.00	1.00	1.00
2.	1.16 (1.00–1.32)	1.08 (0.98–1.19)	1.12 (0.98–1.26)	1.08 (0.98–1.18)
3.	1.25 (1.07–1.45)	1.10 (0.99–1.21)	1.16 (1.02–1.30)	1.09 (0.99–1.20)
4. Most unemployment	1.52 (1.30–1.77)	1.28 (1.16–1.41)	1.35 (1.20–1.52)	1.24 (1.13–1.36)
Percentage reduction in hazard ratio		46%		31%

* Model 1: adjusted for age, model 2: additionally adjusted for education and occupation.

** Percentage reduction calculated as 100*((RRmodel A−RRmodel B)/(RRmodel A−1)) in the quartiles of most unemployment.

Source: Van Lenthe et al (2005). *Journal of Epidemiology and Community Health*, **59**, 223–30 (reprinted with permission).

In the first model among males, the age-adjusted risk in the highest versus the lowest quartile of neighbourhood unemployment was highest in the Whitehall II study (HR = 1.70, 95 per cent CI. 1.22–2.36), and lowest in Turin (HR = 1.28, 95 per cent CI. 1.23–1.35). In model 2, the distribution of education and occupation of the study participants was also taken into account. Adjustment for these compositional factors attenuated the hazard ratio of mortality from 31 per cent in the GLOBE study to 73 per cent in the Whitehall II study. Hazard ratios of living in the 25 per cent neighbourhoods with the highest compared to the lowest unemployment rates remained significantly increased in all studies, except in the Whitehall II study (HR = 1.19, 95 per cent CI. 0.79–1.78). The highest hazard ratios were found in the neighbourhoods with the highest unemployment rates; this pattern was slightly different in the ARIC study. Among females, essentially similar patterns were observed, but due to lower mortality, the estimations were less precise. The age-adjusted hazard ratios were attenuated after adjustment for education and occupation, and remained significantly increased in the ARIC study (HR = 1.63, 95 per cent CI. 1.20–2.22), in Turin (HR = 1.12, 95 per cent CI 1.05–1.20) and Madrid (HR = 1.24, 95 per cent CI 1.13–1.36).

As described, differences in the size of the association could have been expected for several reasons, such as the absolute levels (and ranges in the levels) of deprivation. The large range in unemployment across studies did not allow the examination of categories with similar absolute cut-offs, so percentile-based categories specific to each study were used. This implies that the groups compared may differ by country. It is interesting to note the similarity in hazard ratios in Helsinki and Madrid despite there being large differences in neighbourhood unemployment rates between the two cities. This suggests that the way in which unemployment is distributed across cities influences the hazard of mortality, regardless of the absolute level of unemployment. Second, differences in the size of the associations could have been due to differences in degree of residential segregation by socio-economic position. However, adjustment for education and occupation did not result in substantial country differences in the associations. Such adjustments partly reflect the influence of individual-level socio-economic position on mortality, as well as the influence of residential segregation.

The study showed a similarity in the (size of) associations in different countries. Although it cannot be excluded that different mechanisms are driving these associations between countries, the findings make it tempting to speculate about a general mechanism underlying the associations. For example, it may be the case that an increase or decrease in the neighbourhood socio-economic environment is associated with similar changes in the physical and social neighbourhood environment in all countries. Further, selective migration processes, in which determinants of either wealth or health determine moves and place of residence, could occur across countries. It is also possible that the countries studied were not different enough in policies to allow for the detection of modification of area effects by country.

Increasing understanding of neighbourhood inequalities in health: conceptual and methodological issues

The analyses described above confirm the association between the neighbourhood socio-economic environment and health, and showed a similarity in their size across countries. They show the importance of further exploring the explanations of these inequalities through research. There are several aspects of the studies described above that call for further investigation. Perhaps the first aspect noticed by researchers interested in making a contribution to the explanation of neighbourhood inequalities in health is the lack of conceptual models. As Kaplan recently mentioned: 'Perhaps nowhere is the need for social epidemiological theory more apparent than in the study of place effects on health' (Kaplan 2004). From the findings described above, and using similar experiences from studies on inequalities in health at the individual level, a crude model can be developed. This model describes the general factors involved in the associations, as well as the mechanisms through which they may develop.

Clearly, the model ignores the complexity of all processes potentially operating, but it is useful as a framework for describing (1) how research can advance the understanding, and (2) entry points for policy recommendations to reduce (neighbourhood) inequalities in health. According to the model, there are two main mechanisms through which neighbourhood inequalities in health may develop. First, following the principles of a social causation mechanism, determinants of health may be distributed unevenly by neighbourhood socio-economic environment. These determinants can be individual-level factors (compositional factors), but the collective nature of health in neighbourhoods makes it tempting to presume a role for determinants at the neighbourhood level (contextual factors). For matters of simplicity, a distinction in contextual factors is often made between characteristics of the social and the physical environment. According to the second mechanism, those residing in the neighbourhoods with a lower socio-economic environment may be a selective group of relatively unhealthy persons, and this situation

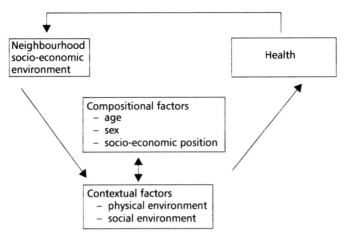

Figure 8.1 A simplified model investigating the association between area deprivation and health.

may be the consequence of migration processes. Similarly, those residing in neighbourhoods with a higher socio-economic environment may be a selective group of relatively healthy persons. For example, those with good health could be more likely to move to more advantaged neighbourhoods, while those with poor health could be more likely to stay in or move to more disadvantaged neighbourhoods.

From the model, four main topics with regard to understanding neighbourhood inequalities in health relate to:

1 The neighbourhood. What is the size of the neighbourhood at which inequalities occur? How do we identify the most deprived neighbourhoods with the poorest health?

2 The mechanisms. What is the evidence for a social causation and selection mechanism in the development of neighbourhood inequalities in health. How can this evidence be improved?

3 The environment. What is the contribution of compositional and contextual factors to neighbourhood inequalities in health? What are the most relevant characteristics of the social and physical environment related to health?

4 The health outcomes. Do neighbourhood inequalities occur in the same direction and magnitude for all health outcomes?

In the remainder of this chapter, important issues related to these questions will be discussed.

The neighbourhood

Defining neighbourhoods

In many studies geographical disparities in health are investigated at the neighbourhood level and in these studies, neighbourhoods are often defined using criteria developed for administrative purposes. The borders of such neighbourhoods do not necessarily overlap with the borders as perceived by the neighbourhood residents; a neighbourhood is not always a synonym for a community and this may have important implications. For example, the strength of the association between social cohesion and health may be larger in neighbourhoods as perceived by residents compared to neighbourhoods based on administrative definitions. This could imply that neighbourhood inequalities in health, as well as the contribution of mediating neighbourhood characteristics, are underestimated if neighbourhoods are defined by administrative criteria. Although for practical (such as the availability of neighbourhood statistics) as well as well for policy reasons, these administrative units will remain measured in studies of neighbourhood inequalities in health, it is important to obtain information on the degree of overlap between objectively defined and subjectively perceived borders of neighbourhoods.

The size of the neighbourhood

At what size of the neighbourhood do inequalities occur? In the study presented earlier in this chapter, the median number of residents ranged from approximately 1.200 to 14.000, yet small and often significant associations between neighbourhood unemployment and mortality were found in all countries examined. The impact of different sizes on the association between the neighbourhood socio-economic environment and poor self-rated health was tested in a Dutch study (Reijneveld *et al.* 2000). In line with our findings, odds ratios of poor self-rated health (and other self-reported health outcomes) for living in the upper compared to the lowest thirds of the neighbourhood socio-economic environment were rather similar for neighbourhoods, postcode sectors (e.g. larger than neighbourhoods), and boroughs.

Although this seems to suggests that within reasonable boundaries, the size of the neighbourhood is not crucially important for the strength of the association between the neighbourhood socio-economic environment and health, a few issues need to be mentioned.

With increasing size of the neighbourhood, there will be an increase in socio-economic heterogeneity of individuals within neighbourhoods. Most likely, neighbourhood inequalities in health will become weaker. Smaller neighbourhoods may result in a more valid measurement of neighbourhood inequalities, but depending on the way the socio-economic environment is measured, measurement error may also increase (Reijneveld *et al.* 2000). One disadvantage of using small and homogeneous neighbourhoods is the inability to study the contribution of factors for which some variation is required, such as residential segregation.

Finally, in selecting neighbourhood units researchers should be guided by theoretical considerations. A key question to be answered before the start of a study is what processes may be mediating the investigated neighbourhood inequalities; a priori expectations about these processes should result in the formulation of hypotheses. For example, if a characteristic of the physical environment is expected to mediate neighbourhood inequalities in a health outcome (for example the availability of sports facilities), the geographical reach of this characteristic determines the area in which residents are exposed to it, and this may guide the construction of the appropriate sizes of the neighbourhoods. Often, several environmental characteristics will contribute simultaneously to neighbourhood inequalities in health, and these characteristics may differ in their reach. While previous multi-level studies often included the individual and neighbourhood level, future studies may need to include more than these two levels.

Measuring the neighbourhood socio-economic environment

For the measurement of socio-economic position at the individual level, there are commonly used indicators (i.e. income, education and occupation), for some of which measurement protocols exist. For the measurement of the neighbourhood socio-economic environment, these factors are less defined. Until now, a wide variety of indicators have been used to describe the neighbourhood socio-economic environment. Among the most often used indicators are the Carstairs and Townsend indices. The latter measures the neighbourhood socio-economic environment by aggregating individual-level data on employment status, occupation, overcrowding, car ownership, and housing tenure to the neighbourhood level. Other studies used data-reduction techniques to construct concepts from a variety of variables. There is no straightforward answer as to how to improve the measurement of the neighbourhood socio-economic environment, but some remarks can be made.

The construction of indicators of the socio-economic environment is often based on the availability of data, as for example in national surveys or in local statistics, and far less on theoretical considerations. More theory seems to be required in the improvement of measures of the socio-economic environment. On the other hand however, translating research findings into policy implications may be enhanced by using routinely collected data in studies on neighbourhood inequalities in health. Further, although integrating elements of the economic, social and physical environment in a single score of neighbourhood deprivation recognizes their mutual dependency it may be useful to disentangle them for the purpose of improving understanding neighbourhood inequalities in health.

Finally, a comparison of neighbourhood inequalities in health using different health indicators is useful for exploring the direction of the processes involved in the development of neighbourhood inequalities in health. There is some evidence that the importance of the choice of the area-level indicator differs by health outcome (Davey-Smith *et al.* 2001). Where the Townsend index of area deprivation seemed to be more strongly related to coronary heart diseases, stroke and stomach cancer, an indicator of social fragmentation was stronger related to suicide mortality.

Mechanisms

The majority of studies on the association between the neighbourhood socio-economic environment and health employ a cross-sectional design. By definition, such studies cannot provide information on causal relationships. Longitudinal studies are required to investigate whether living in poor socio-economic neighbourhood environments subsequently results in poor health, and/or whether selection effects contribute to neighbourhood inequalities in health. Is there evidence for both mechanisms, and how can this evidence be improved?

Selection effects

Neighbourhoods with a low neighbourhood socio-economic environment do not exclusively consist of individuals with a lower individual-level socio-economic position. Depending on the size of the neighbourhood, and on local or national laws and policies, there will be socio-economic heterogeneity in the composition of the neighbourhood residents. Who are the persons with, for example, a higher individual-level socio-economic position residing in neighbourhoods with a low neighbourhood socio-economic environment? At least theoretically it is possible that they are a selective group; an inverse variant of the healthy worker effect (an 'unhealthy resident' effect) may then contribute to neighbourhood inequalities in health via selective migration. According to the mechanism of selective migration, individuals with a higher individual-level socio-economic position, residing in a neighbourhood with a lower neighbourhood socio-economic environment, may live there because their health status required a move to this neighbourhood, prohibited a move to a neighbourhood with a higher socio-economic environment or because their lifestyle (as part of a broader culture) was more consistent with the neighbourhood culture in the lower compared to higher neighbourhood socio-economic environment. Similarly, it cannot be excluded that individuals with a low socio-economic position residing in neighbourhoods with a relatively high neighbourhood socio-economic environment are a selection of individuals with a low socio-economic position with good health. The questions of if, and to what extent, selective migration determines neighbourhood inequalities in health are still largely left unanswered. This may be partly due to the required longitudinal design of studies exploring the process. In a Scottish study, no evidence was found that the probability of limiting long-term illness was higher among migrant groups in the more deprived areas and lower in the less deprived areas (Boyle *et al.* 2002). Preliminary analyses in the Dutch GLOBE study also show that (risk factors of) chronic diseases hardly determine who moves to more deprived or to more affluent areas as compared to those who stay, after taking into account sociodemographic and socio-economic characteristics of individuals (Van Lenthe *et al.* in press). This lack of evidence is in line with a study in which no clear role of selective migration was found in the explanation of urban–rural differences in health (Verheij *et al.* 1998).

Although studies on this mechanism are in line with each other, there is a need for replication of the findings in other studies in order to more firmly refute the mechanism of selective migration. Such longitudinal studies could benefit from including sociological theory as to why persons live where they live; moreover, it seems particularly relevant to focus on the deviant groups, i.e. those who according to their individual level socio-economic position reside in a neighbourhood with either a higher or lower neighbourhood socio-economic environment. As an example, health research related to the transition of living with parents to living independently may be interesting. Where do children with a higher or lower socio-economic position migrate to compared to their parents? It is possible that higher-educated children from parents with a low socio-economic position and a poor health profile have adopted the lifestyle of their parents, and therefore are more willing to stay in neighbourhoods in which these lifestyles are more common. We recently found that the probability of living in neighbourhoods with a relatively low socio-economic environment in adulthood was higher for those with a low socio-economic position in childhood, adjusted for the socio-economic position in adulthood (Monden *et al.* in press). As in other fields of public health research, this implies that understanding selection processes as described above may benefit from adopting a life-course approach.

A causal mechanism

The causal model assumes that the neighbourhood socio-economic environment is related to health via mediating factors, which are related to health and differentially distributed across neighbourhoods of varying socio-economic characteristics. Empirical evidence for a causal model is derived from longitudinal studies among initially healthy populations in which the neighbourhood socio-economic environment can be related to health outcomes during follow-up. An important example providing such empirical evidence comes from data collected in the ARIC Study (Diez Roux *et al.* 2001). After excluding participants with pre-existing coronary heart disease or unknown disease status at baseline, residents of socio-economically disadvantaged neighbourhoods had a higher risk of a coronary heart disease compared to residents in less deprived neighbourhoods in the years after the baseline measurement. In the study, established risk factors of coronary heart disease were also measured at baseline. Adjustment for these risk factors (which to some extent excludes a selection mechanism) did not alter the results substantially.

Another approach to demonstrate a causal model is by linking the neighbourhood socio-economic environment to subsequent changes in health status. For example, living in a poverty area has been associated with a decline in self-perceived health status over a period of nine years (Yen and Kaplan 1999a). Similarly, subjects living in a poverty area showed a greater decline in physical activity as compared to those living in a non-poverty area (Yen and Kaplan 1998).

Currently, the causal mechanism is dominant in thinking about processes underlying neighbourhood inequalities in health over the selection mechanism, but further research is required. Again, the longitudinal study of deviant groups may help to find support for a causal mechanism. A relevant question is to what extent health of individuals with a high socio-economic position changes after moving into neighbourhoods with a poor neighbourhood socio-economic environment. Further, evidence for a causal mechanism could be strengthened by better measurement of exposure to the neighbourhood. It has been suggested that the time spent daily or weekly in neighbourhoods contributes to the difference in neighbourhood inequalities in overweight between men and women, but this needs more empirical support (Van Lenthe and Mackenbach 2002). Similarly, studies may need to include information on the length of the period residents live in a neighbourhood and explore the association between this period and the average health in the neighbourhood.

The environment

The dominance of the causal model is perhaps best reflected by the increasing amount of research examining mediating factors between the neighbourhood socio-economic environment and health. With regard to these mediating factors, distinctions have been made between compositional factors (i.e. age, sex, marital status or socio-economic factors of the neighbourhood residents) and contextual factors (characteristics of the environment). Although this distinction is useful for analytical purposes, it should be noted that these compositional and contextual factors mutually influence each other (MacIntyre et al. 2002). For example, the distribution of play facilities for children may differ between neighbourhoods, with more facilities in neighbourhoods with relatively many families with young children.

A major similarity in most studies on neighbourhood inequalities in health is the substantial reduction in area inequalities in health after adjustment for individual-level socio-economic and sociodemographic factors. With well-known associations between individual-level socio-economic indicators and health, and the increased probability of lower (and higher) socio-economic groups residing in neighbourhoods with a lower (and higher) socio-economic environment, this may come as no surprise. More challenging is the conclusion that remaining parts of the association often could not be explained by these compositional characteristics. Given that health clusters at the neighbourhood level, it is reasonable to assume that contextual factors involved are characteristics of neighbourhoods.

An increase or decrease of the neighbourhood socio-economic environment is not an isolated process; most likely it is a complex process including characteristics of the physical and social environment. Although the notion that health is determined by individual and environmental factors has already existed for some time, the environment has received less attention in public health research in the past decades. Therefore, the question of which environmental characteristics are important for inequalities in health is still largely left unanswered. Yen and Kaplan (1999b) explored the association between aspects of the social environment (including for example the availability of commercial stores and aspects of environment/housing) and 11-year risk of death. The study showed that living in neighbourhoods with a large number of commercial stores or a low housing score (i.e. high population density, low percentage owner-occupied) had an increased risk of death, while the components were only weakly correlated with each other. Studies like these illustrate simultaneously the novelty of this type of research and its complexity. It raises for example the question of which environmental characteristics are relevant for health, the reason this may be so and how to measure them.

To select the most suitable candidate area neighbourhood characteristics, theory from outside the field of public health could be relevant. The association between the neighbourhood socio-economic environment and other characteristics of the neighbourhood has attracted the attention of sociologists, urban geographers and criminologists for some time, but such knowledge has only been introduced moderately in studies of neighbourhood inequalities in health. According to one theory, the neighbourhood socio-economic environment (although in itself determined by a number of factors) may be related to a process of migration, in which the more wealthy persons move out of deprived neighbourhoods, and where the population entering deprived neighbourhoods is characterized by limited financial resources. As most individuals entering neighbourhoods with a poor socio-economic environment do not actively choose these neighbourhoods to live in, they may not intend to stay in the neighbourhood for a long period (Skogan 1990). They may not be inclined to take care of the maintenance of houses and other physical characteristics of the neighbourhood. In these neighbourhoods, it may be less interesting to invest commercially, and existing neighbourhood facilities may disappear. Finally, it is in these neighbourhoods that crime may become more prevalent. Such neighbourhoods may easily enter a spiral of decay, with economical, social and physical deterioration. From a theory like this, potentially relevant factors to be investigated are structural degradation, i.e. a low physical quality of the neighbourhood, a limited availability of neighbourhood facilities and an increased level of crime. Yet this model does not relate these characteristics to health.

MacIntyre and colleagues proposed to start from what humans need in order to lead a healthy life, given the particular socio-economic and sociocultural context (MacIntyre *et al.* 2002). They described a 'hierarchy of human needs', which includes aspects such as air, water and food on the one side and information, personal relationships and play etc. on the other side. From an analysis of basic human needs, measures can be derived and hypotheses about the likely impact of specific features of the local, social and physical environment have to be developed. Identification of environmental characteristics relevant for health may also come from improved ecological models (Sallis and Owen 2002). In these models, the basic assumption is the interaction between the environment and the individual. Existing ecological models are relatively general in nature, but attempts have been made to apply them to specific health outcomes recently, such as for obesity (Swinburn *et al.* 1999).

The physical environment

How can the physical environment contribute to the explanation of neighbourhood inequalities in health? Clearly, there may be a direct pathway between physical characteristics of the neighbourhood and health. Increased air pollution from companies or traffic may affect the health of residents.

The physical environment may also facilitate (or prohibit) healthy behaviour: This can be well illustrated for leisure-time physical activity. The increasing prevalence of physical inactivity in leisure time cannot be entirely due to changes in individual psychosocial factors, such as attitudes. The availability of or distance to sport and recreational facilities may differ for residents of different neighbourhoods of varying socio-economic environments, and there is some evidence of a relationship with physical activity (Sallis *et al.* 1990). Some studies have reported an association between the general physical attractiveness of a neighbourhood and levels of physical activity.

There may also be more indirect pathways between the physical environment and health. It has been shown that the number of billboards with smoking advertisements is higher in more disadvantaged neighbourhoods (Hackbarth *et al.* 1995). Further, physical characteristics may act as stressors and as such influence health via psychosocial factors (Steptoe and Feldman 2001).

Future studies need to include characteristics of the physical environment. Advanced methodological tools such as geographical information systems may help in describing the distribution of these characteristics. Preferably, objectively measured and residents' perceptions of the neighbourhood characteristics should be measured simultaneously.

The social environment

It is well known that social factors at the individual level, such as social support, are beneficial for health. But is there evidence for a role of variables of the social environment at the neighbourhood level? In the past years, an increasing number of studies have concentrated on this question.

Recently, a study found an ecological association between social capital (measured by trust, reciprocity and membership of civic associations) and population mortality at the neighbourhood level (Lochner *et al.* 2003). Among the most important questions is that of whether social capital is a community-level resource (a public good, an ecological characteristic) or an individual-level resource (as a result of membership within social networks). Given an association with health, this has implications for interventions: is it appropriate to develop interventions at the individual or community level?

Other studies have used concepts such as social cohesion, social disorganization and collective efficacy. These concepts have been used in different disciplines, but were only recently introduced in studies of inequalities in population health. Therefore, important gaps remain in knowledge about the contribution of aspects of the social environment for health. First, more knowledge is required about the processes linking the social environment to individual characteristics and ultimately to health. The simultaneous inclusion of social variables at the neighbourhood and individual level may contribute to improved understanding. There is little research that includes individual and neighbourhood level variables of the social environment simultaneously in one study. Second, with regard to the relationship between, for example, social cohesion and health, it should be mentioned that negative health effects cannot be entirely excluded. Third, the measurement of the concepts is still far from being standardized and validated. Different variables may be used to measure the same constructs, while there may be overlap in variables used for different constructs.

Contagion

A specific, and often forgotten neighbourhood characteristic in research is the prevalence of unhealthy behaviour or a disease in neighbourhoods itself. For example, a high percentage of smokers in neighbourhoods may increase the likelihood of young neighbourhood residents starting smoking, while it may reduce the likelihood of smoking cessation. The degree to which such a process of contagion contributes to neighbourhood inequalities in health is yet to be determined from longitudinal studies.

Cross-level interactions

With the distinction made between contextual and compositional variables, it is easy to forget that these variables may interact; the effects of neighbourhood characteristics on health may differ for subgroups and this may provide valuable information for the understanding of neighbourhood inequalities. As a clear example, Stafford and Marmot (2003) hypothesized that individuals with a lower socio-economic position residing in more affluent neighbourhoods would report a relatively poor self-rated health. However, they found no evidence to support this hypothesis.

Future studies will almost certainly aim to investigate a causal mechanism of neighbourhood inequalities in health. With regard to the contribution of characteristics of the physical and social environment, there is a need to advance thinking of the most relevant variables, and to improve measurement methods. With regard to the latter, studies should, for example, explore the relative importance of objective neighbourhood characteristics (as for example measured with geographical information systems) and the same characteristics as perceived by the residents.

Health outcomes

Do neighbourhood inequalities occur for all health outcomes? Investigating and comparing the existence of neighbourhood inequalities for different health outcomes may result in hypotheses about the processes underlying the associations. Several studies investigated neighbourhood inequalities in a variety of biological and behavioural risk factors, and often reported such inequalities in most of these factors (perhaps with the exception of serum cholesterol). A clear example where the physical and social environment may play an important role in the occurrence of neighbourhood inequalities of different outcomes is in the field of injuries. Cubbin *et al.* (2000) showed an inverse relationship between the neighbourhood socio-economic environment and homicide and suicide mortality. It seems likely that different elements of the environment contribute to the occurrence of neighbourhood inequalities for different diseases, and together they may contribute to the reported inequalities in all cause mortality.

In addition, there is evidence that the size and direction of neighbourhood inequalities may be outcome-specific. For example, in epidemiological studies physical activity is often measured by summing leisure time physical activity, occupational physical activity, transport-related physical activity and sport activities. Using these aspects separately and adjusted for individual-level socio-economic position, a higher probability of transport-related physical activity was found in neighbourhoods with a low socio-economic environment and a higher probability of leisure time physical activity was found in more affluent areas (Van Lenthe *et al.* 2005). Similarly, while there was no evidence of neighbourhood inequalities in alcohol consumption in the GLOBE study, among those consuming alcohol the probability of beer consumption was higher in the neighbourhoods with a low socio-economic environment, while the probability of wine consumption was higher among those residing in the neighbourhoods with the highest socio-economic environments (Monden *et al.* in press). It was suggested that these differences could reflect differences in neighbourhood cultures or in material circumstances.

To further understand neighbourhood inequalities in health, specific outcomes seem to be important. For such specific outcomes, it may be less complex to speculate about the processes underlying associations, as well as about the elements of the neighbourhood environment involved in the mechanism.

Conclusions

Two centuries ago, ecological studies showed neighbourhood inequalities in health. Recent multi-level studies confirmed these findings, and showed in addition that both compositional and contextual factors are involved in the processes underlying these inequalities. With a strong focus on health and determinants of health at the individual level in research in the past decades, contemporary studies integrating individual and environmental determinants are confronted with conceptual and methodological problems. In order to improve understanding neighbourhood inequalities in health, theories need to be developed relating neighbourhood socio-economic environment to other neighbourhood characteristics, individual characteristics and ultimately to health and specific health outcomes. Substantial efforts need to be made to identify the most relevant environmental characteristics, and to improve the methodology to measure these characteristics. Inclusion of these characteristics in longitudinal studies, preferably using a life course approach, should result in substantial empirical evidence of the relative contribution of individual and environmental determinants to socio-economic inequalities in health at the individual and neighbourhood level.

Policy implications

There is now substantial evidence of neighbourhood inequalities in health. Moreover, studies have shown that these inequalities are not entirely due to compositional factors, such as age and individual-level socio-economic position of neighbourhood residents. It is likely that elements of the social and physical neighbourhood environment also contribute to neighbourhood socio-economic inequalities in health. What are the entry points for policy recommendations to reduce socio-economic inequalities in health based on these findings?

The first policy implication, even if this is not a novelty, is that neighbourhoods should be used as a setting for interventions aimed at reducing socioeconomic inequalities in health. Neighbourhoods with a low socio-economic environment host relatively many individuals with a low socio-economic position and therefore effective interventions in these neighbourhoods may substantially contribute to the reduction in socio-economic inequalities in health. A second implication of the findings is that both characteristics of individuals and the environment should be the target in such interventions. While targeting individuals is a relatively commonly used approach, improving elements of the living environment with the aim to improve health needs more attention. From the model described in this chapter it can be inferred that relevant improvements may include the neighbourhood socio-economic environment (for example by housing policies aimed at minimizing residential segregation), as well as the related social and physical environment. Environments need to be shaped in such a way that they facilitate health and health-related behaviour, and discourage unhealthy behaviour. Examples of potentially important interventions include increasing neighbourhood facilities, neighbourhood safety and social cohesion. In constructing new neighbourhoods, the health consequences for future residents of the built environment should be taken into account.

It needs to be recognized that improving environmental characteristics in neighbourhoods via policy measures is not easy; it may for example be hampered by competing resources, and by obscurity about responsibilities of residents and professionals. Yet the relationship of environmental characteristics with health may be an argument to intensify efforts of improving the environment in deprived neighbourhoods.

A promising approach in which the neighbourhood is used as a setting for health promotion, and in which interventions are employed at both the individual (compositional) and environmental (contextual) level is the community-based approach. A key principle of the approach is community participation, for example in the development of interventions. Community participation is expected to be of particular importance in order to reach lower socio-economic groups, of whom it is known that they are difficult to reach with traditional health education interventions. A second principle is inter-sectoral collaboration of professionals, which may facilitate interventions on environmental characteristics. Public health professionals, as well as other professionals at the municipal level and local grass roots organizations need to be mobilized, with the aim to build public health capacity across a wide range of stakeholders. Thus far, only a few studies have been carried out to evaluate the effectiveness of community-based interventions in deprived settings. In general, the health effects of these studies were limited and not very consistent (Kloek 2004). This may be due to the fact that there are many chains in these studies, varying from the bottom-up initiation to the final evaluation of projects, and that the strength of the overall effect is as strong as the weakest chain. Currently, the lack of environmental interventions in these studies may be such a weak chain.

In conclusion, health policies aimed at reducing socio-economic inequalities in health should not be confined to individuals and to proximal determinants of health. Almost two centuries after the first ecological studies showed neighbourhood inequalities in health, there is a need and a challenge to include neighbourhood characteristics in interventions and policies aimed at the reduction of socio-economic inequalities in health.

Acknowledgement

Although parts of this chapter express the view of the author, I am indebted to all members of ESF Working Group 3 (Macrosocial determinants of morbidity and mortality: their contribution to the explanation of inequalities in health) for sharing thoughts over the past years. I would like to thank specifically Ana Diez-Roux, Luisa Borell, Mai Stafford, Pekka Martikainen, Timo Kaupinnen, Tapani Valkonen, Chiara Marinacci, Giuseppe Costa and Enrique Regidor for their contribution to the analyses presented in this chapter. Part of this chapter is reproduced from a paper published in the *Journal of Epidemiology and Community Health* (2005, **59**, 223–30), with permission from the BMJ Publishing Group.

References

Borell L, Diez Roux AV, Rose K, Catellier D, Clark BL (2004). Neighbourhood characteristics and mortality in the Atherosclerosis Risk in Communities Study. *International Journal of Epidemiology*, **33**, 398–407.

Bosma, H, Mheen DH van de, Borsboom GJJM, Mackenbach JP (2001). Neighborhood socio-economic status and all-cause mortality. *American Journal of Epidemiology*, **153**, 363–71.

Boyle P, Norman P, Rees P (2002). Does migration exaggerate the relationship between deprivation and limiting long term-term illness? A Scottish analysis. *Social Science and Medicine*, **55**, 21–31.

Cardano M, Costa G, Demaria M (2004). Social mobility and health in the Turin longitudinal study. *Social Science and Medicine*, **58**, 1563–74.

Cubbin C, LeClere FB, Smith GS (2000). Socioeconomic status and injury mortality: individual and neighbourhood determinants. *Journal of Epidemiology and Community Health*, **54**, 517–24.

Davey-Smith G, Whitley E, Dorling D, Gunnell D (2001). Area-based measures of social and economic circumstances: cause-specific mortality patterns depend on the choice of index. *Journal of Epidemiology and Community Health*, **55**, 149–50.

Diez Roux AV, Stein Merkin S, Arnett D, *et al.* (2001). Neighbourhood of residence and incidence of coronary heart disease. *New England Journal of Medicine*, **345**, 99–106.

Haan M, Kaplan GA, Camacho T (1987). Poverty and health. Prospective evidence from the Alameda County Study. *American Journal of Epidemiology*, **125**, 989–98.

Hackbarth DP, Silvestri B, Cosper W (1995). Tobacco and alcohol billboards in 50 Chicago neighborhoods: market segmentation to sell dangerous products to the poor. *Journal of Public Health Policy*, **16**, 213–30.

Kaplan G (2004). What's wrong with social epidemiology and how can we make it better? *Epidemiologic Reviews*, **26**, 124–35.

Kloek GC (2004). Improving health-related behaviour in deprived neighbourhoods. Erasmus MC Rotterdam, PhD-thesis.

Lochner KA, Kawachi I, Brennan RT, Buka SL (2003). Social capital and neighborhood mortality rates in Chicago. *Social Science and Medicine*, **56**, 1797–805.

MacIntyre S, Ellaway A, Cummins S (2002). Place effects on health: how can we conceptualise, operationalise and measure them? *Social Science and Medicine*, **55**, 125–39.

Mackenbach JP, Mheen Hvd, Stronks K (1994). A prospective cohort study investigating the explanation of socio-economic inequalities in health in the Netherlands. *Social Science and Medicine*, **38**, 299–308.

Marinacci C, Spadea T, Biggeri A, Demaria M, Caiazzo A, Costa G (2004). The role of individual and contextual socio-economic circumstances on mortality: analysis of time variations in a city of north west Italy. *Journal of Epidemiology and Community Health*, **58**, 199–207.

Marmot MG, Davey-Smith G, Stansfeld S *et al.* (1991). Health inequalities among British civil servants: the Whitehall II study. *Lancet*, **337**, 1387–93.

Martikainen P, Kaupinnen T, Valkonen T (2003). Effects of the characteristics of neighbourhoods and the characteristics of people on cause specific mortality: a register based follow-up study of 252 000 men. *Journal of Epidemiology and Community Health*, **57**, 210–17.

Monden CWS, Lenthe FJ van, Mackenbach JP (in press). Neighbourhood and childhood socio-economic environment, self-assessed health and health-related behaviours: the GLOBE study. *Health and Place*.

Picket K and Pearl M (2001). Multilevel analyses of neighbourhood socio-economic context and health outcomes: a critical review. *Journal of Epidemiology and Community Health*, **55**, 111–22.

Regidor E, Gutierrez-Fisac JL, Calle ME, Navarro P, Dominguez V (2002). Infant mortality at time of birth and cause-specific adult mortality among residents of the Region of Madrid born elsewhere in Spain. *International Journal of Epidemiology*, **31**, 368–74.

Reijneveld SA, Verheij RA, Bakker DH de (2000). The impact of area deprivation on differences in health: does the choice of the geographical classification matter? *Journal of Epidemiology and Community Health*, **54**, 306–13.

Ross NA, Wolfson MC, Dunn JR *et al.* (2000). Relation between income inequality and mortality in Canada and in the United States: cross-sectional assessment using census data and vital statistics. *British Medical Journal*, **320**, 898–902.

Sallis JF, Hovell MF, Hofstetter CR *et al.* (1990). Distance between homes and exercise in facilities related to the frequency of exercise among San Diego residents. *Public Health Reports*, **105**, 179–85.

Sallis JF and Owen N (2002). Ecological models of health related behaviour. In: K Glanz, BK Rimer BK, FM Lewis (eds) *Health behaviour and health education*, pp. 462–84. Jossey-Bass, San Francisco, CA.

Skogan W (1990). *Disorder and decline: crime and the spiral of decay in American neighborhoods*. University of Berkely, Berkely, CA.

Slogett A and Joshi H (1994). Higher mortality in deprived areas: community or personal disadvantage? *British Medical Journal*, **309**, 1470–4.

Stafford M and Marmot M (2003). Neighbourhood deprivation and health: does it affect us all equally? *International Journal of Epidemiology*, **32**, 357–66.

Stafford M, Martikainen P, Lahelma E, Marmot M (2004). Neighbourhoods and self-rated health: a comparison of public sector employees in London and Helsinki. *Journal of Epidemiology and Community Health*, **58**, 772–8.

Steptoe A and Feldman P (2001). Neighbourhood problems as sources of chronic stress: development of a measure of neighbourhood problems, and associations with socio-economic status and health. *Annals of Behavioural Medicine*, **23**, 177–85.

Swinburn B, Egger G, Raza F (1999). Dissecting obesogenic environments: the development and application of a framework for identifying and prioritising environmental interventions for obesity. *Preventive Medicine*, **29**, 563–70.

The ARIC investigators (1989). The Atherosclerosis Risk in Communities (ARIC) Study. *American Journal of Epidemiology*, **129**, 687–702.

Townsend P and Davidson N (1982). *Inequalities in health: The Black Report.* Penguin, Harmondsworth.

Van Lenthe FJ and Mackenbach JP (2002). Neighbourhood deprivation and overweight: the GLOBE study. *International Journal of Obesity*, **28**, 664–83.

Van Lenthe FJ, Borell LN, Costa G *et al.* (2005). Neighbourhood unemployment and all-cause mortality: a comparison of six countries. *Journal of Epidemiology and Community Health*, **59**, 223–30.

Van Lenthe FJ, Martikainen P, Mackenbach JP (in press). Neighbourhood inequalities in health and health-related behaviour: Results of selective migration. *Health and Place*.

Van Lenthe FJ, Brug J, Mackenbach JP (2005). Neighbourhood inequalities in physical inactivity: the role of neighbourhood attractiveness, proximity to local facilities and safety. *Social Science and Medicine*, **60**, 763–75.

Verheij R, Mheen D van de, Bakker DH de, Groenewegen PP, Mackenbach JP (1998). Urban–rural variations in health in the Netherlands: does selective migration play a role? *Journal of Epidemiology and Community Health*, **52**, 487–93.

Veugelers P, Yip A, Kephart G (2001). Proximate and contextual socio-economic determinants of mortality: multilevel approaches in a setting with universal health care coverage. *American Journal of Epidemiology*, **154**, 725–32.

Villermé L (1826). Rapport fait par M. Villermé, et lu à l'Académie royale de Médicine, au nom de la Commission de statistique, sur une série de tableaux relatifs au movement de la population dans les douze arrondisement municipaux de la ville de Paris, pendant les cinq années 1817, 1818, 1819, 1820 et 1821. *Archives of General Medicine*, **10**, 216–47.

Yen IH and Kaplan GA (1998). Poverty area residence and changes in physical activity level: evidence from the Alameda County Study. *American Journal of Public Health*, **88**, 1709–12.

Yen IH and Kaplan GA (1999a). Poverty area residence and changes in depression and perceived health status: evidence from the Alameda County Study. *International Journal of Epidemiology*, **28**, 90–94.

Yen IH and Kaplan GA (1999b). Neighborhood social environment and risk of death: multilevel evidence from the Alameda County Study. *American Journal of Epidemiology*, **149**, 898–907.

Chapter 9

Welfare state regimes and health inequalities

Espen Dahl, Johan Fritzell, Eero Lahelma,
Pekka Martikainen, Anton Kunst and
Johan P. Mackenbach

Introduction

This chapter is motivated by an empirical finding that has led to much confusion, namely that in the Western, industrial hemisphere relative health inequalities seem about as large in egalitarian countries as in the less egalitarian ones (Mackenbach *et al.* 1997, 2003, Kunst *et al.* 1998 a, b, 2005). This puzzling and challenging evidence is the topic for our chapter. In order to impute meaning to this phenomenon, we will attempt to link two strands of research, comparative welfare state research and comparative research on health inequalities. Until now, these two research areas have developed separately almost in total isolation form each other, but we believe that comparative health inequality research would benefit from being informed by recent advances in comparative welfare state research, and vice versa.

After years of research and debate, there is a general agreement that the way in which societies are organized can have important effects on the health of populations in general and health inequalities in particular. Yet it is highly uncertain which macro-social factors are the most influential. We will investigate macro-social factors that are held to be relevant for health inequalities and that are related to welfare and health policies, socio-economic policies, welfare state institutions and the socio-economic outcomes of these factors. The Nordic, or Scandinavian countries, i.e. Denmark, Finland, Norway and Sweden, are of special interest in this respect. The generic term for welfare arrangements in the four Nordic countries is the Social Democratic welfare state model (Erikson *et al.* 1987, Esping-Andersen 1990, 1999). This model is characterized by egalitarian institutional features that are shown to produce egalitarian outcomes. Thus, according to established knowledge, the Nordic countries are expected to have generally high levels of average health and smaller social inequalities in health.

Over the past decade, several studies have been carried out with the aim to assess whether the Nordic welfare states indeed have achieved a relatively narrow health gap between disadvantaged groups and other sections of the population. The results from various studies are not consistent. Some were quite unexpected and suggested larger inequalities in the Nordic countries than elsewhere. These results raised debates on both methodological issues and substantial interpretations. Yet it remains unclear what these results imply for the Nordic welfare state model. A closer inspection and careful interpretation of the empirical findings is needed before one can address the question of whether the Nordic welfare state model can be regarded as a positive example of how health inequalities depend on the way in which society is organized.

In the chapter we proceed as follows: we begin by re-evaluating the reasons one might have to expect that some welfare states regimes, and especially the Nordic one, can be expected to influence inequalities in population health. The welfare state research literature will be evaluated by addressing the following questions: (a) What are the main characteristics of different welfare state regimes? (Special attention will be paid to the welfare state regimes model of Esping-Andersen (E-A) (1990, 1999).) (b) What social consequences are these different regimes expected, and demonstrated, to have? (c) What consequences may be expected for inequalities in health? Guided by these questions, we will review the themes, core ideas and research findings of recent welfare states research.

We will go on to assess whether the expected effects of welfare state regimes were observed in recent research on inequalities in health. We will review the empirical evidence brought forward by recent comparative studies. Special attention is given to comparative studies on health inequalities that include both Nordic countries and countries with different welfare state regimes. Most of this research deals with 'traditional' inequalities between socio-economic groups, but we will also consider 'new' inequalities by focusing on selected disadvantaged groups for whom empirical evidence is available, such as lone mothers. When reviewing the evidence, we will discuss methodological issues as these need to be treated carefully when exploring the effects of welfare state regimes. One key issue is the difference between relative and absolute inequalities.

Reflecting on these findings, we will then attempt to determine the potential importance of welfare states for health inequalities. Our findings will show whether or not different welfare state regimes are associated with different levels of social inequalities in health. A predictable finding is that social inequalities in health do persist in Nordic countries as well as elsewhere. Does this finding imply that welfare state institutions are relatively unimportant, as compared to other factors (e.g. culture, history) that underlie social inequalities in health? Or can a particular role of welfare state regimes be discerned, perhaps in combination with some other factors? A reflection on these issues will be made on the basis of a careful assessment of comparative empirical data on welfare state regimes and on health inequalities.

Welfare state regimes

Over the last decades, social scientists have provided a number of categorisations of welfare states (for an overview see Midgley 1997, Abrahamson 1999, Kautto *et al.* 2001). Titmuss (1974) made a distinction between 'three contrasting models or functions of social policy' (Lødemel and Trickey, 2001). These were developed to analyse differences in welfare state provision, and the ideas and ideologies of the role of the state underlying them. The first, The Residual Model of Welfare, sees the function of social services as one of dealing only with people who are unable to help themselves. The second, The Handmaiden Model, rests on the view that social services are functional to other institutions, that 'social needs should be met on the basis of merit, work performance and productivity'. The Institutional Redistributive Model 'sees social welfare as a major integrated institution in society, providing universalistic services outside the market on the principle of need'.

However, it was not until the publication of E-A's (1990) exceptionally influential *The three worlds of welfare capitalism*, that the work and discussion of typologies became mainstream in comparative research. The basic claim was that we cannot understand welfare state variation linearly but that there are qualitative differences in the way social provision is provided and that welfare states tend to cluster into three different regimes forming interconnected configurations of state and market, and later, the family. He distinguishes between three ideal types of welfare state *regimes*, defined according to two dimensions: extent of decommodification, i.e. the extent to which social policy make individuals independent of the market, and stratification and labour market participation, i.e. the extent to which the welfare state differentiates in the treatment of different groups. Esping-Andersen identified three 'worlds of welfare states', which he labelled 'conservative-corporatist', 'liberal', and 'social-democratic' regimes. The first is characterized by strong emphasis on the role of social partners, on the principle of subsidiarity, and in consequence on an underdeveloped service sector and on the existence of labour market 'insiders' and 'outsiders'; and empirically it is illustrated for example by France and Germany. The second is characterized by minimal and targeted assistance measures, re-enforcement of job-seeking behaviour and promotion of systems of private welfare provision, and is illustrated by the UK and the US. The third idealized type, the 'social-democratic' regime, exemplified by the Nordic or Scandinavian countries, is characterized by institutionalized redistribution, where the welfare state provides universal social rights, based on full employment (Esping-Andersen 1990).

The actual criteria for this classification are based on information on institutional features of the social security arrangements in each country in the 1980s. The defining criteria are degree of universalism and generosity of social security programmes such as unemployment benefits, pension insurance and sickness pay. Because such programmes are expensive, the Nordic model is based on the premise of full employment, since its sustainability relies on a broad tax base. Thus, pertaining to this model are also features like relatively high employment rates, including among women and the elderly, and active labour market policies (Huber and Stephens 2001). Although not one of E-A's defining criteria, the social democratic welfare states are also characterized by a big public sector that to a large degree is occupied by women.

One logical derivation of the Nordic welfare state design is that these societies would be characterized by a low degree of social inequality. This expectation is confirmed: a large body of empirical evidence shows that the Nordic welfare states enjoy a high level of social equality. For example, numerous analyses based on the Luxembourg Income Study (LIS), probably the best database on comparative income and poverty studies, indicate that income inequality (measured by the Gini index) is consistently lower in these countries than in most others. The same applies to poverty: poverty rates among people in their working ages, as well as poverty rates among vulnerable groups such as the elderly and single mothers, are low compared to nations in the other welfare regimes (Atkinson 2000, Fritzell 2001, Smeeding 2002).

The 'power resources' school (Korpi 1983) maintains that the Nordic model received its particular form through 'class compromises' forged between the labour movement, first in alliance with agrarian interests, and later in coalition with the middle classes and their political organizations. The result is that basic social benefits are not only universal and comparatively generous, but are also earnings-related reflecting differences in work and earnings records. Therefore everyone, both the haves and the have-nots, has an objective interest in maintaining the welfare state. The fact that an institutional structure that also supports the well-off has been comparatively successful in fighting poverty was phrased 'the paradox of redistribution' by Korpi and Palme (1998).

E-A's regime typology served as the backdrop for most comparative welfare state studies that were conducted throughout the 1990s and up until today. We will deliberately omit commenting upon the rather fruitless debate on how many welfare regimes that can be differentiated because the Nordic countries tend to cluster together in all suggested typologies. Here we will limit ourselves to four comments on this huge body of literature which are most relevant to our research questions.

Criticism of Esping-Andersen's typology

Narrow focus on income maintenance and the old industrial worker family

The actual operationalization of welfare in E-A's notion of 'welfare regime' is rather narrow. As mentioned, the defining criteria are related to potentials for decommodification in social security programmes. This implies that important welfare benefits and in particular welfare services are left out, such as child care, education, elderly and health care. In theory, these welfare institutions may have profound influences on health and health inequalities. On the other hand, all the countries embedded in the Nordic cluster score medium to high on both child care, education and health care expenses, and all have universal health insurance founded on the principle of equal access (Rostgaard and Lehto 2001; Gornick and Meyers 2003; Huber and Stephens 2001). Moreover, in an attempt to distinguish social care models Anttonen and Sipilä (1996) concluded that there was a common Nordic model.

Regimes are gender blind

A major criticism that was raised against E-A's 'three worlds' was that the analysis was gender blind, and if the welfare of women and families was considered, the picture of regime types would have been different (Orloff 1993). The first part of this argument is certainly true, but the second is not. E-A himself took this critique seriously and has responded to it (Esping-Andersen 1999). Here, he accepted that his initial analysis lacked a gender/family perspective, so he extended the scope by focusing on the changing role of women, for example by studying family policies and additional welfare outcomes such as fertility rates. His main conclusion was that with respect to family policies, his original typology would fit neatly. Countries with social democratic regimes have also developed family-friendly polices that are more or less absent in the other two regimes. These policies allow women to combine their roles as mothers, spouses and workers more smoothly than elsewhere (Esping-Andersen 1999).

Regimes are outdated

Some have argued that institutional changes that took place during the 1990s have altered the nature of the Nordic welfare state architecture. Gilbert (2002) maintains that over the past decades Western countries have witnessed a paradigmatic shift in welfare provision which he conceptualizes as the enabling state. This concept emerges out of empirical comparisons of international data indicating a general move 'toward work-oriented policies, privatisation of social welfare, increased targeting of benefits and the shift from an emphasis on the social rights of citizenship to the civic duties of community members' (Gilbert 2002 p. 5). However, the comparative evidence, the interpretation of this evidence and its causes and social consequences are all matters of dispute (Beckfield 2003). More specifically, as for the Nordic countries, the vast majority of all serious research efforts suggest that the Nordic model is still fairly distinct (see e.g. Kautto *et al.* 2001; Swank *et al.* 2002; Huber and Stephens 2001). By and large this was also the conclusion from the elaborated work of the large research commission that was appointed to describe trends in living conditions in Sweden in the 1990s (Palme *et al.* 2002). Possible social consequences of recent welfare reforms are addressed next.

Rising inequality in the Nordic countries?

Has social inequality become more widespread and grown deeper in the Nordic countries, as some claim? In Finland, Norway and Sweden, it appears that income inequality increased during the 1990s, but this increase came about during the second half of the 1990s at a time when the economy was booming. Still, there is hardly any convincing evidence that social inequality more generally soured dramatically during the 1990s as a whole, and income inequality in the Nordic countries is still among the lowest in the world. Moreover, business cycles affected the Scandinavian countries differently during the 1990s. No other Western countries underwent such severe economic crisis in the early 1990s as Finland and Sweden. Finland especially was hit hard by the collapse of trade with the Soviet Union. Finland's experience is particuary remarkable since despite the external shock it neither cut welfare spending substantially nor developed higher income inequality or increased poverty (Kautto *et al.* 1999, 2001). In Norway and in Denmark the voyage was smoother through these turbulent years.

Collecting the threads, we have attempted to make the case that the four Nordic countries form a rather homogeneous welfare state cluster with certain unique institutional features that are expected to, and indeed proven to be favourable to social equality, and that these features, by and large, prevail today.

Implications for health inequalities

Before we start developing hypotheses about possible links between welfare regimes and health inequalities, we will clarify what we mean by 'social inequalities in health'. First, the social part – or more accurately the socio-economic part – may include different dimensions of social stratification like wealth, power and prestige, often operationalized as income, social (or occupational) class, education, and occupational prestige. In this chapter we will primarily, but not exclusively, focus on occupational class. Second, with respect to inequalities there is an important distinction between the absolute and relative dimension. Relative measures are calculated by dividing, for example, rates of ill-health among people with high and low social status. Absolute inequalities are calculated by subtracting rates of ill-health among people with high and low social status. Division and subtraction will not necessarily produce the same results, especially if the levels of ill-health and survival between countries or regimes differ, which they often do. Clearly there is more than mathematics involved in this, and we will pursue this issue in the discussion section.

Why and how should welfare regimes influence health inequalities? When attempting to formulate hypotheses about this, we can distinguish between two approaches, one holistic and one atomistic.

A holistic approach would imply a view that the regime as a whole is what really matters, i.e. the entire and unique configuration of family, state and markets pertaining to each type. It is not so much the specific, but the general feature that drives the clockwork. The general evidence supporting this holistic perspective is small inequalities in a wide variety of social outcomes. Health inequalities, like other kinds of inequalities, are influenced by societal conditions in general. An atomistic approach implies asking what are the particular qualities of the Nordic welfare model that would serve as mechanisms to further a comparatively egalitarian health outcome. Elaborating the latter strategy, we will spell out five possible links informed by, on the one hand E-A's typology and on the other hand insights from health inequality research.

1 Universalism, social integration and health inequalities

2 Decommodification, preservation of health and health inequalities

3 Public benefits and services, equal access and use and health inequalities

4 A strong labour movement, good working conditions and health inequalities

5 Welfare state institutions, the life course and health inequalities.

Universalism, social integration and health inequalities

Universalism means that welfare benefits and services are granted to everyone on the basis of citizenship. In his classic essay, Marshall (1950) puts heavy emphasis on social citizenship as a 'natural' expansion of civil and political rights in Western societies. The implications of universalism may be profound. It means that before the Government every citizen is of equal worth despite prevailing class inequalities, everyone is entitled to social services and (material) benefits, and on these equal terms everyone is included in the society. It is a reasonable hypothesis that universalism has a larger potential to include all citizens than the two other welfare regimes. Thus universalism may foster social integration, social cohesion, social capital, a general support for the welfare state and a sense of belonging among all citizens, also among the less privileged groups. Assuming that social integration and social capital, and hence 'good feelings' and less antisocial behaviour are beneficial for health (Wilkinson 1996), universalism would bring about better health and smaller health inequalities than other welfare regimes.

Comparative research supports the view that regimes influence the well-being of the citizens and attitudes that indicate social capital. Rothstein and Steinmo (2002) show that key social capital indicators like trust and membership in voluntary organizations have higher levels in Sweden than in other countries; Putnam (1999) demonstrates that levels of trust are higher in the Nordic countries than in other welfare states. Polls show that there is a high degree of support of the core institutions of the welfare state (Huber and Stephens 2001), but also that there are regime-specific variations: Linos and West (2003) demonstrate that cross-country differences in the social bases of support for redistribution confirm predictions of welfare state regimes. Andress and Heien (2000) show that 'range of governmental action' (as measured by three variables measuring attitudes to reduce income differences, provide jobs for all, and basic income for all) vary by welfare state regime (which the authors label 'cultural integration') as one might expect, and also by regime-specific economic interests and socialization. Taken together, this evidence indicates that different welfare state regimes do fertilize social capital and public attitudes, i.e. 'culture', in ways that might affect health inequalities in the direction assumed.

Decommodification, preservation of health and health inequalities

The concept of decommodification draws attention to the opportunities for 'all' citizens to opt out of work and still be able to maintain the material means to lead a decent life. It thereby creates protection from fierce market forces. Along with universality, generosity is a major ingredient of decommodification: everyone is covered, and when covered they can go on with the life they are accustomed to. Under such circumstances most people do not have to fear selling their house, their belongings, or losing their job if health fails. This is also likely to dampen the potentially health-threatening effects of stressful life events like unemployment and might engender a feeling of social security and protection from the 'risk society'. This protection also means freedom: freedom to choose to work or to choose not to work when the circumstances are difficult. In turn, this freedom to choose would probably foster a sense of control over the circumstances of life. In the psychosocial model, (a feeling of) control over the future is an essential salutogenetic factor (Elstad 1998). With a sense of security and a sense of control come psychological well-being and probably also good mental and physical health. Again, compared to the less privileged in other welfare regimes, these features should be of particular importance to the disadvantaged in the Nordic countries and thereby reduce health inequalities (see Chapter 7).

Traditionally, the Nordic welfare states have had high employment rates, and, despite the recession of the 1990s, still have in comparison to other countries (Esping-Andersen 2002). The model is actually based on this premise, not necessarily because it is good for individuals, but because it is a precondition for the survival of the entire sociopolitical system. A likely side-effect of high employment rates is better health. Since unemployment is related to poorer health, this characteristic would predict narrower health inequalities (Martikainen and Valkonen 1996, Warr 1987, Iversen and Sabroe 1988, Lahelma 1992, Keefe *et al.* 2002).

Decommodification may also influence health inequalities through a different and more straightforward mechanism, i.e. by granting employees the opportunity to withdraw from work for shorter or longer periods of time because of ill-health. Blue collar workers and lower salaried employees are in greater need of such opportunities than higher salaried employees for at least three reasons. First, their health is generally worse; second their physical and psychosocial work environment is poorer, less secure, more demanding, and less rewarding and supportive; and third their ability to cope with a stressful and demanding work environment tend to be lower thus creating a higher level of vulnerability to stress (Hallqvist *et al.* 1998, Marmot *et al.* 1999). Groups with lower occupational status tend to experience job strain and imbalance between effort and reward more often than do higher ranked occupational groups. In light of this, it comes as no surprise that sickness rates among lower ranked employees are consistently higher than among higher ranked employees (Marmot *et al.* 1999). Generous sick pay schemes ensure that sick workers can withdraw from work and yet maintain their living standards, at least for some time. This aspect of decommodification may benefit the health and well-being of the individual as well as the society in that it promotes high employment rates among groups with poorer health, i.e. women, the elderly, and lower socio-economic groups. Inasmuch as such welfare arrangements allow groups with lower occupational status to attend to their health, they will also contribute to smaller health inequalities (Kivimäki *et al.* 2003).

Public benefits and services, equal access and use and health inequalities

In the contemporary debate on macro-social determinants of health inequalities, Wilkinson (1996) and others emphasize the importance of social capital and social cohesion. In opposition to this interpretation, neo-materialists highlight the role of politics, social investments and social infrastructure. In these accounts, the Nordic welfare states are expected to produce good population health, and probably also small health inequalities (Coburn 2000, Navarro *et al.* 2003). Certainly, the Nordic welfare states have a rich provision of publicly financed welfare and health services that in principle are equally accessible for all. In terms of public expenditures on health care, social care and public benefits, the Nordic countries are all among the high spenders in Europe. From a neo-materialist perspective, these characteristics lead us to expect smaller health inequalities.

Strong labour movement, good working conditions and health inequalities

The labour movements have made a salient imprint on the social democratic welfare societies and it is likely that this extends into the workplace. Recent evidence suggests that characteristics of the workplace are important for health and health inequalities (Elstad 2003). On the one hand, highly developed local democracy at the workplace, advanced work environment legislation, and a high degree of unionization mean that all workers, including blue-collar workers, have their say. Surveys indicate that overall, workers in the Nordic countries have relatively favourable working conditions (Paoli and Merllié 2001). It also seems reasonable to suggest that in the Nordic welfare states blue-collar workers in relative terms have a better physical and psychosocial work environment; e.g. they fare better on job strain (Karasek and Theorell 1990), on the effort–reward imbalance instrument (Siegrist 1996), and also regarding physical working conditions, exposures to chemical and biological health hazards and ergonomic problems, although such problems do prevail in the Nordic countries (Dahl and Elstad forthcoming). We do not know whether unskilled workers in social democracies fare better than their counterparts in the other regime types relative to white-collar workers, but based on an assessment of power of the labour movement to influence social-democratic societies over the past 70 years or so, and the social institutions that are established, our (hopefully qualified) guess is that the working conditions among unskilled workers are relatively decent.

Welfare state institutions, the life course and health inequalities

It is claimed that the Nordic welfare state is there for you from the cradle to the grave. If so, this should have a bearing on the life course approach to health inequalities. This points to risk exposures, health hazards and social disadvantages in early life that may have long-term effects into adult life (see Chapter 2 in this book). Approaches in this perspective are biological imprint in early life that may have long-term influences on health, accumulation of good or bad social circumstances, exposures and behaviours, and social and biological pathways. Comparatively low rates of child poverty indicate that this may be a less severe problem in later years than elsewhere (Fløtten 1999) although we cannot dismiss the possibility of long-term effects on the health status of today's elderly of more widespread and deeper poverty before the Second World War. Very low infant mortality rates testify to the view that living conditions and health care are of high quality, although social inequalities in infant mortality have not been eradicated (Arntzen 1993, Östberg 1996). Comprehensive arrangements of medical rehabilitation, activation measures and opportunities for education and life-long learning suggest that unfortunate life events like job loss and impaired health may have less severe consequences for well-being and life chances than elsewhere. Welfare and health services may be more effectively geared towards breaking vicious circles of accumulated social problems and risks. Of particular interest is the adolescent/adult transition, which is assumed to be particularly influential regarding both later socio-economic conditions and health (West 1991). The fact that higher education is paid collectively suggests that the adolescence–adult transition may be smoother in the social-democratic welfare states than in other regimes.

We have attempted to make the case that health inequalities will be smaller in social democratic than the conservative and the liberal regime types. Our next question is: What does the evidence reveal?

A review of the European evidence on health inequalities

In this section, we review the European comparative evidence on the patterns and magnitude of health inequalities in mortality and morbidity, contrasting the different welfare state regimes, the Nordic-social democratic, the liberal and the traditional-conservative. Our main focus is the comparison between the Nordic countries and those belonging to the two other regimes.

Health inequalities in Europe: cross-sectional evidence

Mortality

International comparative research on inequalities in mortality and morbidity began to accumulate from the late 1970s onwards (Karisto *et al.* 1978, Valkonen 1989). One of the first European comparisons included six countries and examined educational inequalities in mortality in the 1970s (Valkonen 1989): the study showed that the lower the level of education, the higher the mortality. The Nordic countries had neither particularly small or large inequalities. Instead the association was very similar in all countries, with men having a steeper gradient than women.

An EU-funded project including 11 European countries compared inequalities in mortality in the 1980s (Mackenbach *et al.* 1997, Kunst 1997, Kunst *et al.* 1998a). The socio-economic indicator was social class, and differences between manual and non-manual male workers were compared. Relative inequalities in mortality in the 1980s were largest among French middle-aged men, followed by Finnish men: The smallest inequalities were found in Denmark, Norway and Italy. Educational differences in mortality were also studied in a smaller set of countries. This analysis confirmed that France and Finland had large inequalities; and Italy was also among the countries with large inequalities (Kunst and Mackenbach 1994).

However, looking at absolute inequalities in mortality the picture is not exactly the same as that for relative inequalities (Kunst 1997, Vågerö and Erikson 1997, Kunst *et al.* 1998b, see also Lundberg and Lahelma 2001, Lundberg 2003). In Table 9.1 we have presented results from a selection of countries to demonstrate how the picture of inequality and rank order of the countries vary by measure of health inequality. The figures are borrowed from Lundberg (2003) who used data from the EU projects.

Three features of Table 9.1 are worth noting. First, the social democratic country, Sweden has comparatively large relative inequalities in mortality, but has small absolute inequalities. The reason for this switch in the rank order is the overall low mortality level in the country and that Swedish white-collar workers in particular have exceptionally low mortality. Second, another social democratic country, Finland, has large relative as well as absolute inequalities. These are larger than those of a liberal regime country like England and Wales. By implication there are substantial differences in mortality within the social democratic camp. Third, the conservative representative in Table 9.1, France, has the highest relative as well as absolute occupational inequalities in mortality.

Table 9.1 Relative and absolute differences in occupational mortality among men aged 45–65 years of age. Mortality risks among blue collar versus white-collar workers in selected countries.

	Relative inequality	**Absolute inequality**
Social democratic regime		
Denmark	1.33	5.2
Norway	1.33	6.3
Sweden	1.40	5.6
Finland	1.52	9.8
Conservative regime		
France	1.70	11.5
Liberal regime		
England and Wales	1.45	7.5

Sources: Kunst *et al.* (1998), Lundberg (2003).

Morbidity

Analyses of inequalities in self-rated health by education in the 1980s found that *relative* health inequalities tended to be particularly large in three Nordic countries – Denmark, Norway and Sweden – and average in Finland (Mackenbach *et al.* 1997, Cavelaars *et al.* 1998a). Analysing differences in morbidity by occupational class confirmed that these inequalities were not smaller in the Nordic countries than elsewhere in Europe (Cavelaars *et al.* 1998c). Countries such as Germany, Spain and Italy, belonging to the liberal and the traditional-conservative regime had smallest health inequalities by education and occupational class among men. However, inequalities seemed to depend on the socio-economic indicator, as further analyses on income inequalities in self-rated health showed a somewhat different picture: Finland and Sweden had average level of inequalities and Germany again the narrowest (Cavelaars *et al.* 1998b, Mackenbach *et al.* 2005). In the Nordic countries health inequalities by income were smaller than those by education as compared with other countries. As mentioned, this may reflect the fact that the Nordic countries have smaller income inequalities than other European countries (Atkinson *et al.* 1995). Largest health inequalities by income were found for British and Dutch men, and British women.

The finding that inequalities in morbidity do not vary systematically between welfare state regimes may suggest that within Europe the different welfare regimes are not divergent to the extent that they produce clear and distinct patterns of health inequalities. A comparison of health inequalities including employees from Britain, Finland and Japan provides a case in point. Japan represents a vastly different and mixed cultural background including traditional eastern and modern Western elements. Nevertheless, its welfare state regime can be said to be more traditional conservative than any of the European countries (Martikainen *et al.* 2004). Among men from all of the three countries, as well as British and Finnish women, an expected Western pattern of health inequalities was found, with upper white-collar employees having the best health and the manual class the worst. However, Japanese women classified by their own occupational class showed little evidence of the Western pattern of health inequalities. Thus, strongly contrasting welfare state regimes may also show contrasting relative health inequalities, and this may concern women in particular. Gender-segregated patterns of labour force participation and welfare provision within different welfare regimes may be associated with different patterns of health inequalities, as exemplified by the case of Japanese employed women.

For morbidity we have to rely on relative inequalities only since reliable and comparable data on absolute levels and socio-economic differences of morbidity across different countries are unavailable. Judging from the relative inequalities in morbidity we can conclude, first, that overall these inequalities do not show systematic differences between countries belonging to different welfare state regimes. Second, however, inequalities in morbidity are likely to vary by the socio-economic indicator. While educational and occupational class inequalities in morbidity tend to be large in the Nordic countries, the inequalities by income tend to be average, possibly due to small income inequalities per se.

Lone mothers

Socioeconomic inequalities in health may be modified by marital and parental status and this is more likely among women than men (Arber and Lahelma 1993). In particular, lone mothers constitute a disadvantaged group among women. Accordingly a stream of research on multiple roles and health has examined the influence of marital and parental status as well as employment status on women's health (Arber and Khlat 2002). The effects of lone motherhood on health may be due to stress, adverse material circumstances, or selection into lone motherhood on the basis of health degrading characteristics. In particular lone mothers' position provides a case of health inequalities which has been studied in a number of countries. Despite this, rigorous comparative analyses on the health of lone mothers are still rare.

Lone motherhood has been associated with mortality and morbidity in numerous studies (Martikainen 1995, Ringbäck *et al.* 2000) in the Nordic countries and in the UK and these associations have been shown to be largely independent of socio-economic status. A study comparing Britain and Finland (Lahelma *et al.* 2002a) found that employed women with children had the best health measured by limiting long-standing illness and self-rated health in both countries, while lone mothers overall had the poorest health. Similar findings were obtained in a study comparing Britain and Sweden (Whitehead *et al.* 2000, Burström *et al.* 1999). A further study comparing women's health in Finland and Sweden found that in both countries lone mothers who were not employed were at a particular high risk of poor health (Roos *et al.* 2005).

Summarizing the comparative evidence suggests that the mortality and morbidity of lone mothers is approximately equally poor in Finland and Sweden, Nordic regime countries, as in Britain, a liberal regime country. However, in Britain the poor health of lone mothers is due to their disadvantaged socio-economic and labour market position. In the Nordic regime countries social policies have encouraged women combining motherhood and paid employment, and this is likely to have supported lone mothers' socio-economic and material position. However, thus far it is difficult to assess whether the high mortality and morbidity of lone mothers is independent of selection on the basis of other characteristics. Overall the excess poor health of employed lone mothers is relatively modest, but being the additional factor of unemployment is associated with high risk of morbidity and mortality.

Health inequalities in Europe: evidence on trends

Changes over time in health inequalities may tell a different story than the cross-sectional patterning of health, and different determinants may lie behind the differences per se and their trends. While a broad range of factors from historical to current circumstances contribute to the cross-sectional patterns and magnitude of health inequalities, rapid cultural and structural changes, economic upheavals and policy shifts may also contribute to changes in health inequalities.

Mortality

Socioeconomic inequalities in mortality in six national settings among the middle aged were compared from the early 1980s to the mid 1990s (Mackenbach *et al.* 2003). The overall trend was towards widening relative inequalities in all the countries studied. However, absolute inequalities remained fairly stable, except in Finland where even absolute inequalities widened. This widening was, first of all, due to faster mortality decline from cardiovascular diseases in the higher socio-economic groups. Additionally, increasing rates of lung cancer and breast cancer among women with low education and injuries, contributed to the widening as well (Valkonen *et al.*

2000). The Nordic countries present a fairly mixed picture. In four Nordic countries higher-status men showed a clear decline in mortality, which was less rapid among men with lower socio-economic status. Also lower educated Norwegian and Danish women showed less favourable trends, since their mortality stagnated over the studied period. Along the same lines, Swedish data reveals that women with unskilled manual worker position have a stagnating mortality risk over the 1980s and 1990s. Among British men the trends in inequalities in mortality were very similar to Nordic men.

Thus an overall widening in relative inequalities in mortality has occurred since the early 1980s. No consistent differences between the welfare state regimes can be observed, and there is considerable heterogeneity among the Nordic countries. Gender seems to have a bearing on changes in inequalities in mortality in some Nordic countries, with lower status women's mortality stagnating. However, due to lack of data on women from other European countries it is not yet possible to say whether similar trends can be found among women elsewhere.

Morbidity

Socioeconomic inequalities in morbidity were compared in ten European countries from the 1980s to the 1990s (Kunst *et al.* 2005). Although there is much uncertainty due to insufficient data, the overall trend suggests widening inequalities in morbidity which may be somewhat stronger among women than men. The results suggest the largest widening for Italy and Spain. In the Nordic countries the trends in inequalities in morbidity may be somewhat more stable than elsewhere in Europe.

These findings are supported by a couple of other comparative studies. A Nordic survey found a stable tendency in health inequalities from the 1980s to the 1990s (Lahelma *et al.* 2002b). This finding is all the more important since Sweden and particularly Finland underwent a deep economic recession with high rates of unemployment in the early 1990s. However, the downturn was not followed by widening health inequalities in either country. Furthermore, changes over time in health inequalities in Britain and Finland over the same period suggested contrasting trends: in Finland health inequalities remained stable or tended to narrow slightly, whereas in Britain they remained stable or tended to widen (Lahelma *et al.* 2000).

Taken together, the comparative evidence from available studies suggests that inequalities in morbidity over time may have remained more stable in the Nordic welfare states than in other European countries. In Sweden and Finland this still held true during a strongly adverse economic climate in the early 1990s. It can be suggested, but remains largely an open question, that these trends indicate that the Nordic welfare state regime with its relative high levels of social benefits and services serve as a buffer against adverse structural changes (Kunst *et al.* 2005, Lahelma *et al.* 2002b).

Unemployment, recession and mortality

Unemployment is a stressful life-event with potential repercussion for health. The harmful effects of recession on the well-being and health of individuals are also potentially modified or buffered by welfare policies.

Previous observational follow-up studies of individuals have shown that mortality rates among the unemployed are higher than among the employed (Moser *et al.* 1984, Iversen *et al.* 1987, Morris *et al.* 1994), and high morbidity among unemployed is widely documented (Warr 1987, Dooley *et al.* 1996). The association between health and unemployment may be due to the causal effects of unemployment or to a greater risk of unemployment among those with a greater risk of future ill-health and mortality. The effects of unemployment on mental well-being are fairly well established and concern Nordic countries as well as other European countries (Warr 1987, Iversen and Sabroe 1988, Lahelma 1992, Keefe *et al.* 2002). However, the causal effects of unemployment on severe physical ill-health are less well known.

The deep recession in Finland in the early 1990 is a useful context in which to assess the contribution of unemployment on health (Martikainen and Valkonen 1996, Lahelma *et al.* 2002b). Overall these studies indicate that the effects of recession on mortality and morbidity seem to be modest; the declining trend in mortality continued unaffected. No adverse changes were observed in groups that can be considered particularly vulnerable, such as the unemployed or less educated.

However, it is unclear whether the small effects of the recession on health trends are due to policy interventions by the welfare state. Alm (2001) presents one longitudinal study supporting such a view in that she found that the health consequences of unemployment were much smaller among those unemployed people who were covered by the unemployment insurance system. Still, long-term trends in physical ill-health that are related to unhealthy behaviours may be relatively insensitive to unemployment in the first place, and thus short-term economic shocks may be small as compared to long-term secular changes in health behaviours. No comparative evidence to assess these possibilities exists.

Summary and discussion

Based on the theoretical and empirical literature on welfare state regimes, we formulated five propositions as to why we expected health inequalities to be smaller in social democratic regimes than in the conservative and the liberal regime clusters. Our review of the available empirical evidence shows that health inequalities are found in all countries, among men as well as women. The magnitude of these inequalities varies, but does not consistently reflect the different welfare regimes; also within the social democratic camp we find marked heterogeneity. For example, with respect to occupational inequality in mortality measured in relative terms, Denmark and Norway are ranked among the countries with lowest inequality while Sweden is in the middle and Finland is among the countries with the highest inequality. In absolute terms, Norway and Sweden have the lowest inequality, Denmark is in the middle and Finland again has high inequality. One qualification of this is that the size of the inequalities varies by socio-economic indicator: occupational differentials in health appear larger than income inequalities in some social democratic welfare states. Comparative data on trends suggest that inequalities in health over time may have remained more stable in the Nordic welfare states than in other European countries. In Sweden and Finland this held true even during a strongly adverse economic climate in the early 1990s. This might indicate that the social democratic welfare state regime, with its relatively high levels of social benefits and services, has the potential to buffer against adverse economic shocks (Kunst *et al.* 2005, Lahelma *et al.* 2002b).

In sum, available evidence shows that health inequalities are not consistently, significantly and systematically smaller in the social democratic countries than in countries belonging to the two other welfare regimes, i.e. the conservative and the liberal.

We will address this finding by discussing problems with data and statistical measures, the welfare state regime typology and the propositions we have derived, and the possible importance of unanticipated and undesired side effects of welfare state institutions.

Data and measures

Mortality data from the social democratic regime countries are of better quality than that from countries belonging to other regimes. This is because in the Nordic countries mortality is linked to census/register information on occupation, education and income by means of personal identification number for the entire population. Less random or systematic noise in the data in social democratic countries may make the statistical associations more accurate (Lundberg and Lahelma 2001). On the other hand, survey data are hardly of better quality than those collected elsewhere in Europe and because of comparatively small sample sizes in the Nordic countries, the data often have less statistical power. What further complicates comparisons of inequalities in self-reported health measures is the fact of unmeasured differences in cultural definitions of health and illness and readiness to report (ill-) health. These phenomena will probably vary considerably between countries and, even more importantly, between the same social groups between countries. Hardly anything is known about how such social and cultural influences may bias the results.

Comparison of nominally similar socio-economic positions across countries is also difficult. An educational level such as 'lower secondary' may represent entirely different levels of knowledge and socio-economic prospects in one country compared to another. Similarly, even though much effort has been made to develop and apply common social class schemes in many European countries (Cavelaars *et al.* 1998c), a class such as 'unskilled manual worker' does not represent an identical social group in different countries. Such difficulties can only partly be resolved by the use of statistical techniques, such as those based on relative instead of absolute measures of socio-economic status. This is inherent to cross-country comparisons: while differences between countries make these comparisons of interest, the same differences imply that the constructs used do not have identical meanings. One should therefore be cautious in interpreting health inequalities between countries and over time.

An important issue is the way in which 'inequality' is measured in the available comparative studies. For example, we lack measures that are sensitive to different population sizes in different socio-economic groups across countries, regimes and over time. Because welfare policies in different regimes may aim at changing the entire social structure differently, e.g. different policies to enhance social mobility among people in the lowest and most vulnerable social positions, this kind of information should be taken into account in empirical analyses of health inequalities. However, comparative studies that included health equality indices which took into account distributions of people across socio-economic levels (e.g. the Index of Dissimilarity; measures comparing income quintiles) did not observe a consistently better position of Nordic countries either (Kunst 1997; Kunst *et al.* 2005).

For some Nordic countries, e.g. Sweden, it matters significantly whether one bases the comparisons on absolute or relative inequalities. The explanation is partly mathematical (as may easily be demonstrated): the mortality level is extremely low in Sweden. This makes it 'hard' to achieve narrow relative health inequalities in this country. Thus, Sweden will be 'punished' if one relies only on relative measures and completely ignores absolute ones. It is hard to justify that an overall low level of mortality poses a problem. However, the issue of whether relative or absolute measures should be used is more than one of mathematics. It involves scientific, public health and philosophical aspects.

From a scientific and explanatory point of view, relative measures are the most informative by revealing the deeper social processes that generate health inequalities. From a public health and health policy point of view, absolute measures may be more informative for the assessment of the achievements of the welfare state in general and health policies in particular.

Philosophically, one might argue that neither relative nor absolute comparisons of inequality in health are sufficient. A third comparison should also be made, namely that of the mortality level among the worst off in different countries. Lundberg and Lahelma (2001) have pointed out that manual workers in Sweden have the lowest mortality rate in the European countries from which data exist. From a philosophical perspective, this is an important piece of information: Rawls claims that a society should be judged on the basis of how the worst-off fare. As discussed by Lundberg (2003) assuming that manual workers are the worst off in Rawls' sense, this means that a rational actor would pick Sweden as their home country when placed behind the 'veil of ignorance'. The judgement of how fair a society is cannot exclusively or predominantly be based on the well-being of groups that are better off in a particular society. Comparisons across societies are also indispensable. As many commentators now seem to agree, relative comparisons should be complemented with absolute measures. In addition, we would argue, comparisons of health and mortality levels among the worst off in different countries should also be made.

This discussion does not apply to Finland which has high relative as well as absolute inequalities in mortality signifying that there are large differences in health inequalities within the social-democratic camp. This issue is difficult to tackle within the regime typology of E-A and it suggests that a number of secular trends and other factors may be at work which may not necessarily be closely intertwined with the welfare state development per se, but which nevertheless may contribute to health inequalities. First, demographic trends, such as urbanization and family formations, including cohabitation and single households also potentially impact on health inequalities. Second, some structural developments, such as the increase in educational attainment, may be largely independent of welfare state regimes. Third, the impacts of past living conditions are extended upon current conditions as well. This can be seen for example in the differential development of health inequalities by birth cohort in different Nordic countries. In Finland inequalities in morbidity in older birth cohorts are larger than in the other Nordic countries, whereas in younger cohorts such differences between countries are no more visible (Silventoinen and Lahelma 2002). Given that Finland is a latecomer in the Nordic welfare regime (Kangas 1991, Alestalo and Flora 1994), we would expect such a result and also that inequalities in mortality in Finland gradually will resemble the pattern we find in the three other Nordic countries.

Counteracting forces?

The evidence indicating that our propositions fail to receive convincing support may be interpreted in several ways. One is that the welfare state of the Nordic type also generates unanticipated and undesired side-effects on the health status among low status people. To a certain degree these forces offset the benign processes generated by the welfare state. We can speculate on three such mechanisms, the 'bowling alone' syndrome, relative deprivation, and class related consumption patterns.

The *bowling alone* metaphor is borrowed from Putnam (1999) who used the phrase to describe the erosion of social capital, i.e. mutual trust, social participation and reciprocity, in the USA over the past 30 years. One reinterpretation of the argument in this context draws attention to the possibility that state welfare undermines civic society, social capital, and informal social networks and communities. This critique of the welfare state of the social democratic type goes against most theorising on welfare regimes and empirical evidence: as we saw earlier, all empirical findings on social capital, e.g. trust, membership in voluntary organizations, and public opinions towards the welfare state suggest that the Nordic countries do very well in this are. Based on this evidence this is hardly an important factor.

Relative deprivation may have an ambiguous effect on health inequalities. Wilkinson (1996) argues that social systems characterized by large income inequalities suffer from high degrees of relative deprivation and poorer health. In its original tap the notion of relative deprivation was formulated to explain the paradoxical empirical finding that open opportunity structures caused dissatisfaction among subgroups of people competing for social rewards, i.e. that soldiers who had the best training and education were more dissatisfied with their pace of promotion, even if they advanced more rapidly than others (Stouffer *et al.* 1949). Relative deprivation stems from expectations and comparisons with significant others. These social processes will unfold in all social systems where inequality is present, and in welfare states like the Nordic ones: one could even speculate that the Nordic welfare states, with their egalitarian ethos and social structures, create a high level of frustration and stress because they generate high levels of expectation of upward social mobility and prosperity among the less privileged – expectations that are seldom met (Åberg Yngwe *et al.* 2003). This line of reasoning leads to the hypothesis that health inequalities would also be marked in Nordic welfare states, and may be particularly visible in stress-related conditions: heart disease for example. We do acknowledge, however, that this is a speculative argument.

Socio-economic differences in smoking prevalence seem to be particularly high in the Nordic countries (Cavelaars *et al.* 2000, Giskes *et al.* 2005) as are differences in mortality from heart disease (Mackenbach *et al.* 2000). Thus, it might be that a causal link between socio-economic position and health is partly mediated by *health-related behaviours*. The question is why groups with lower socio-economic status are more inclined to consume and behave in ways that are detrimental to health in the Nordic countries than elsewhere in Europe. One speculative answer is that they can afford it because of fairly high minimum wages and universal and comparatively generous benefits. If so, the question immediately becomes why these groups *choose* to spend their money on unhealthy consumption. Part of the answer might be that these countries are in a more mature phase of the smoking epidemic, and many who started decades ago have become addicted, for example. Another and related answer is that most if not all public health education and health campaigns focusing on smoking, drinking, diets, and exercising tend to be universal and directed towards to all citizens. It is likely that higher socio-economic groups respond more readily to these messages and are more willing and able to change their health-related behaviour accordingly. Thus, this mass strategy may lead to the unintended (and undesired) consequence that relative health inequalities increase, although public health in general may improve.

We have seen welfare institutions mainly as causal forces. Perhaps a more fruitful approach is to look at them as buffers. Comparative data indicate that widening overall trends in inequalities in morbidity as well as mortality can be found in Western Europe (Lahelma *et al.* 2002b, Kunst *et al.* 2005, Mackenbach *et al.* 2003). However, it appears that changes over time in health inequalities may vary by the type of welfare state regime. There are suggestions of stable inequalities in morbidity in Finland and Sweden in the early 1990s despite a deep economic recession. Simultaneously, non-Nordic countries showed more widening inequalities in morbidity during periods in which the economic situation was stable. Whether this relatively weak evidence suggests that the social democratic regime, with its broader welfare state arrangements, may help buffer against adverse conditions that generate health inequalities remains nevertheless an open question. We suggest that regimes may also matter for relative health inequalities, but perhaps more like buffer mechanisms than as prime causal mechanisms.

Health-related social and occupational mobility might not be a major determinant of health inequalities in general, but could it play a more pronounced role in the Nordic countries than elsewhere in Europe? Although we have stressed that comparative research has documented that the Nordic countries have small social inequalities, comparative research on social mobility rather underlines commonality across nations. Erikson and Goldthorpe (1992, 2002) emphasize that no Western nation stands out as having markedly more inter-generational social fluidity, i.e. relative rates of mobility, than others. Overall, as indicated by the title, *The Constant Flux*, changes over time and differences in social mobility between Western countries are small. It should be noted, however, that their research deals solely with inequality of opportunity rather than inequality of outcome, e.g. health, and few truly comparative studies of social mobility have focused on health as a driving force, i.e. health-related social mobility (Rahkonen *et al.* 1997).

Nordic welfare states show comparatively low levels of inequalities for many social outcomes, income being one of the most prominent. However, it is harder to redistribute health than to redistribute money. By nature health is not like income or other material/tangible goods: income is divisible while health is not. Unlike income one cannot redistribute health directly; a piece of health cannot be transferred from a rich person to a poorer, at least not on a large scale (although the new transplantation technology might prove other-wise in the future). Thus (re)-distribution of health cannot be achieved by the means by which social democratic welfare states usually redistribute income, i.e. by public transfers and progressive taxation. Despite this inherent differ-ence between the two goods, health and e.g. income, it does not mean that welfare arrangements are impotent in influencing the distribution of health. Rather, it means that the welfare state must do so in an indirect way, that is, by modifying the determinants – be they behavioural, social or structural – of health. In terms of political opportunities, the difference between income and health is one of degree and not one of principle: it is almost impossible to influence the social distribution of health in a direct way, but not in an indirect way, by changing the health determinants.

Over the past few decades research on health inequalities has focused on inequality as social stratification and not inequality conceived of as poverty, social exclusion, or as occupying a marginal, disadvantaged position. Vulnerable, disadvantaged groups may include lone mothers, long-term unemployed, long-term poor, certain immigrant groups, and recipients of social assistance. The scanty comparative research on such groups is more or less limited to lone mothers. As mentioned, the health status of this group in Scandinavian countries is similar to that in other European countries. Perhaps the health status of disadvantaged and vulnerable groups such as these should also be in focus when evaluating the performance of different welfare regimes? Such comparative evidence is lacking.

There are several white spots on the map that are worthy of deeper exploration in the future. Let us point out four. First, there is a need for *improving data* and making them comparable. Second, more research is needed on the five possible *mechanisms* linking regimes to health inequalities, for example those related to universalism, decommodification, and free or cheap public services. Third, in addition to studying social stratification, researchers should also initiate comparative studies of the health of *disadvantaged groups* such as lone mothers and long-term unemployed. Fourth, we need more comparative research on *health-related social mobility* in different countries, especially studies focusing on mobility into and out of the labour market.

Conclusion

Available evidence shows that health inequalities are not consistently, significantly and systematically smaller in the social democratic countries than in countries belonging to the two other welfare regimes, i.e. the conservative and the liberal. However, for inequalities in mortality except for Finland the other Scandinavian countries do perform rather well, in relative terms (Denmark and Norway) or in absolute terms (Norway and Sweden). The 'deviant' Finnish case calls for looking for other forces and mechanisms, for example related to long-term effects of a poor past and a rather young welfare state as well as steep inequalities in cardiovascular and accidental mortality. Data on time trends suggest that social democratic welfare institutions may buffer against detrimental effects of economic recessions.

A cautionary note must be applied here. The sample of countries is somewhat limited. Although the findings are based on the best empirical evidence available, a number of methodological problems remain, among them national differences in how data are collected and processed, the comparability of health measures, and the comparability of socio-economic indicators.

Acknowledgements

The inspiration to write this paper grew out of the discussions that took place in Working Group III: 'Macro-social determinants of morbidity and mortality: Their contribution to the explanation of inequalities in health' of the Social Variations in Health Expectancy in Europe Programme funded by the European Science Foundation. The members of this network have contributed much in forming our views on these issues. We would also like to express our gratitude to Professor Vicente Navarro and the editors of this book for their valuable comments on earlier drafts of this chapter.

References

Åberg Yngwe M, Fritzell J, Lundberg, O Diderichsen F and Burström B (2003). Exploring relative deprivation: is social comparison a mechanism in the relation between income and health? *Social Science and Medicine*, 57, 1463–73.

Abrahamsson P (1999). The welfare modelling business. *Social Policy and Administration*, 33, 394–415.

Alestalo M and Flora P (1994). Scandinavia: welfare states in the periphery – peripheral welfare states? In: M Alestalo E Allardt A Rychard W Wesolowski (eds) *The transformation of Europe*, pp. 53–73. *Social Conditions and Consequences*. IFIS Publishers, Warszawa.

Alm S (2001). *The resurgence of mass unemployment. Studies on social consequences of joblessness in Sweden in the 1990s*. Swedish Institute for Social Research, Stockholm.

Andress HJ and Heien T (2000). Four worlds of welfare state attitudes? A comparison of Germany, Norway, and the United States. *European Sociological Review*, 17, 337–56.

Antonen A and Sipilä J (1996). European social care services: is it possible to identify models? *Journal of European Social Policy*, 6, 87–100.

Arber S and Khlat M (eds) (2002). Social and economic patterning of women's health in a changing world. *Special issue of Social Science and Medicine*, 54.

Arber S and Lahelma E (1993). Class inequalities in women's and men's health: Britain and Finland compared. *Social Science and Medicine*, 37, 1055–68.

Arntzen A, Magnus P and Bakketeig LS (1993). Different effects of maternal and paternal education on early mortality in Norway. *Paediatric and Perinatal Epidemiology*, 7, 376–86.

Atkinson AB (2000). Is rising income inequality inevitable? A critique of the transatlantic consensus. 1999 WIDER Annual Lecture, UNU/WIDER, Helsinki.

Atkinson AB, Rainwater L and Smeeding TM (1995). *Income distribution in OECD countries*. OECD Social Policy Studies No. 18. Paris, OECD.

Beckfield J (2003). Review of transformation of the welfare state: the silent surrender of public responsibility. *Social Forces 82*.

Burström B, Diderichsen F, Shouls S and Whitehead M (1999). Lone mothers in Sweden: trends in health and socio-economic circumstances, 1979–1995. *Journal of Epidemiology and Community Health*, 53, 750–6.

Cavelaars A, Kunst A, Geurts J et al. (1998a). Differences in self reported morbidity by educational level: a comparison of 11 Western European countries. *Journal of Epidemiology and Community Health*, 52, 219–27.

Cavelaars A, Kunst A, Geurts J et al. (1998b). Differences in self-reported morbidity by income level in six European countries. In: Cavelaars A. (ed.) *Cross-national comparisons of socio-economic differences in health indicators*, pp. 49–66. Erasmus University, Rotterdam.

Cavelaars A, Kunst A, Geurts J et al. (1998c). Morbidity differences by occupational class among men and women in seven European countries: an application of the Erikson-Goldthorpe social class scheme. *International Journal of Epidemiology*, 27, 222–30.

Cavelaars AE, Kunst AE, Geurts J et al. (2000). Educational differences in smoking: international comparison. *British Medical Journal*, 320, 1102–7.

Coburn D (2000). Income inequality, social cohesion and the health status of populations: the role of neo-liberalism. *Social Science and Medicine*, 51, 135–46.

Dahl E and Elstad JI (forthcoming) *Class Work and Health – Norwegian Country Chapter*. Book chapter submitted to the Winner project.

Dooley D, Fielding J and Levi L (1996). Health and unemployment. *Annual Review of Public Health*, **17**, 949–65.

Elstad JI (1998). The psycho-social perspective on social inequalities in health. *Sociology of Health and Illness*, **20**, 598–618.

Elstad JI (2003). Livsstil, arbeidsmiljøbelastninger og helseulikheter blant 55-årige menn, Tidsskrift for Den norske lægeforening, **123**, 2289–91.

Erikson R and Goldthorpe J H (2002).Intergenerational inequality. A sociological perspective. *Journal of Economic Perspectives*, **16**, 31–44.

Erikson R and Goldthorpe JH (1992). *The constant flux. A study of class mobility in industrial societies*. Clarendon Press, Oxford.

Erikson R, Hansen EJ, Ringen S and Uusitalo H, eds. (1987). *The Scandinavian model. Welfare states and welfare research*. ME Sharpe, New York.

Esping-Andersen G (1990). *The three worlds of welfare capitalism*. Polity Press, Oxford.

Esping-Andersen G (1999). *Social foundations of postindustrial economies*. Oxford University Press, Oxford.

Esping-Andersen G (2002). *Why we need a new welfare state*. Oxford University Press, Oxford.

Fløtten T (1999). *Fattigdom i Norge. Problem eller bagatell?* Fafo-report 303, Oslo.

Fritzell J (2001). Still different? Income distribution in the Nordic countries in a European comparison. In: M Kautto, J Fritzell, B Hvinden, J Kvist and H Uusitalo (eds) *Nordic welfare states in the European context*, pp. 18–41. Routledge, London.

Gilbert N (2002). *Transformation of the welfare state. The silent surrender of public responsibility*. Oxford University Press, Oxford.

Giskes K, Kunst AE, Benach J, *et al.* (2005). Trends in smoking behaviour between 1985 and 2000 in nine European countries by education. *Journal of Epidemiology and Community Health*, **59**, 395–401.

Gornick JC and Meyers MK (2003). *Families that work. Policies for reconciling parenthood and employment*. Russel Sage Foundation, New York.

Hallqvist J, Diderichsen F, Thorell T, Reuterwall C, Ahlbom A, SHEEP Study Group (1998). Is the effect of job strain on myocardial infarction risk due to interaction between high psychological demands and low decision latitude? Results from Stockholm Heart Epidemiology Program (SHEEP) *Social Science and Medicine*, **46**, 1405–16.

Huber E and Stephens JD (2001). *Development and crisis of the welfare state. Parties and policies in global markets*. The University of Chicago Press, Chicago, IL.

Iversen L, Andersen O, Andersen PK, Cristoffersen K, Keiding N (1987). Unemployment and mortality in Denmark. *British Medical Journal*, **295**, 879–84.

Iversen L and Sabroe S (1988). Psychological well-being among unemployed and employed people after a company closedown: a longitudinal study. *Journal of Social Issues*, **44**, 141–52.

Kangas O (1991). *The politics of social rights. Studies on the dimensions of sickness insurance in OECD countries*. Swedish Institute for Social Research, Stockholm.

Karasek R and Theorell T (1990). *Healthy work: stress, productivity and reconstruction of working life*. Basic Books, New York.

Karisto A, Notkola V and Valkonen T (1978). Socio-economic status and health in Finland and the other Scandinavian countries. *Social Science and Medicine*, **12C**, 83–8.

Kautto M, Fritzell J, Hvinden B, Kvist J and Uusitalo H (eds) (2001). *Nordic welfare states in the European context*. Routledge, London.

Kautto M, Heikkilä M, Hvinden B, Marklund S and Ploug N (eds) (1999). *Nordic social policy*. Routledge, London.

Keefe V, Reid P, Ormsby C, Robson B, Purdie G and Baxter J (2002). Serious health events following involuntary job loss in New Zealand meat processing workers. *International Journal of Epidemiology*, **31**, 1155–61.

Kivimäki M, Head J, Ferrie JE, Shipley MJ, Vahtera J and Marmot MG (2003). Sickness absence as a global measure of health: evidence from mortality in the Whitehall II prospective study. *British Medical Journal*, **327**, 364–70.

Korpi W (1983). *The democratic class struggle*. Routledge, London.

Korpi W and Palme (1998). The paradox of redistribution and the strategy of equality: welfare state institutions, inequality and poverty in the Western countries. *American Sociological Review*, **63**, 661–87.

Kunst A (1997). *Cross-national comparisons of socio-economic differences in mortality*. Erasmus University, Rotterdam.

Kunst A and Mackenbach J (1994). The size of mortality differences associated with educational level in nine industrial countries. *American Journal of Public Health*, **84**, 932–7.

Kunst A, Bos V, Lahelma E *et al.* (2005). Trends in socio-economic inequalities in self-assessed health in 10 European countries. *International Journal of Epidemiology*, **34**, 295–305.

Kunst AE, Groenhof F and Mackenbach JP (1998b). Mortality by occupational class among men 30–64 years in 11 European countries. EU Working Group on Socioeconomic Inequalities in Health. *Social Science and Medicine*, **46**, 1459–76.

Kunst AE, Groenhof F, Mackenbach JP and the EU Working Group on Socioeconomic inequalities in health (1998a). Occupational class and cause-specific mortality in the middle-aged men in 11 European countries. *British Medical Journal*, **316**, 1636–41.

Kunst AE, Bos V, Lahelma E, Bartley M *et al.* (2005). Trends in socio-economic inequalities in self-assessed health in 10 European countries. *International Journal of Epidemiology*, **34**, 295–305.

Lahelma E (1992). Unemployment and mental well-being: elaboration of the relationship. *International Journal of Health Services*, **22**, 261–74.

Lahelma E, Arber S, Rahkonen, Silventoinen K (2000). Widening or narrowing inequalities in health? Comparing Britain and Finland from the 1980s to 1990s. *Sociology of Health and Illness*, **22**, 110–36.

Lahelma E, Arber S, Kivelä K, Roos E (2002a). Multiple roles and health among British and Finnish women: the influence of socio-economic circumstances. *Social Science and Medicine*, **54**, 727–40.

Lahelma E, Kivelä K and Roos E *et al.* (2002b). Analysing changes of health inequalities in the Nordic welfare states. *Social Science and Medicine*, **55**, 609–25.

Levitas R (1998). *The inclusive society? Social exclusion and New Labour*. MacMillan Press, Hampshire.

Linos K and West M (2003). Self interest, social beliefs, and attitudes to redistribution. Readdressing the issue of cross-national variation. *European Sociological Review*, **19**, 393–409.

Lødemel I and Trickey H (2001). '*An offer you can't refuse*'. Policy Press, Bristol.

Lundberg O (2003). Ojämlikhet i hälsa: Definitioner, mått, mekanismer och policyimplikationer. *Socialmedicinsk tidsskrift*, **80**, 200–8.

Lundberg O and Lahelma E (2001). Nordic health inequalities in the European context. In: M Kautto, J Fritzell, B Hvinden, J Kvist and H Uusitalo (eds) *Nordic Welfare States in the European context*, pp. 42–65. Routledge, London.

Mackenbach J, Bos V and Andersen O *et al.* (2003). Widening inequalities in mortality in western Europe. *International Journal of Epidemiology*, **32**, 830–7.

Mackenbach J, Cavelaars A, Kunst A, Groenhof F and the EU Working Group on Socioeconomic Inequalities in Health (2000). Socioeconomic inequalities in cardiovascular disease mortality. An international study. *European Heart Journal*, **21**, 1141–51.

Mackenbach J, Kunst A, Cavelaars A, Groenhof F, Geurts J and the EU Working Group on Socioeconomic Inequalities in Health. (1997). Socioeconomic inequalities in morbidity and mortality in Western Europe. *Lancet*, **349**, 1655–9.

Mackenbach JP, Martikainen P, Looman CW, Dalstra JA, Kunst AE and Lahelma E (2005). The shape of the relationship between income and self-assessed health: an international study. *International Journal of Epidemiology*, **34**, 286–93.

Marmot MG, Siegrist J, Theorell T and Feeney A (1999). Health and the psychosocial environment at work. In: MG Marmot and R Wilkinson (eds) *Social determinants of health*, pp. 105–31. Oxford University Press, Oxford.

Marshall TH (1950). *Citizenship and social class and other essays*. Cambridge University Press, Cambridge.

Martikainen P (1995). Women's employment, marriage, motherhood and mortality: a test of the multiple role and role accumulation hypotheses. *Social Science and Medicine*, **40**, 199–212.

Martikainen P and Valkonen T (1996). Excess mortality of unemployed men and women during a period of rapidly increasing unemployment. *Lancet*, **348**, 909–12.

Martikainen P, Lahelma E, Marmot M, Sekine M, Nishi N and Kagamimori S (2004). A comparison of socio-economic differences in physical functioning and perceived health among male and female employees in Britain, Finland and Japan. *Social Science and Medicine*, **59**, 1287–95.

Midgley J (1997). *Social welfare in a global context*. Sage Publications, Thousand Oaks, CA.

Morris JK, Cook DG and Shaper AG (1994). Loss of employment and mortality. *British Medical Journal*, **308**, 1135–9.

Moser KA, Fox AJ and Jones DR (1984). Unemployment and mortality in the OPCS Longitudinal Study. *Lancet*, **2**, 1324–9.

Navarro V, Borrell C, Benach J, Muntaner C *et al.* (2003). The importance of the political and the social in explaining mortality differentials among the countries of the OECD, 1950–1998. *International Journal of Health Services*, **33**, 419–94.

Orloff AS (1993). Gender and the social rights of citizenship: the comparative analysis of gender relations and welfare states. *American Sociological Review*, **58**, 303–28.

Östberg V (1996). *Social structure and children's life chances. An analysis of child mortality in Sweden*. Swedish Institute for Social Research, Stockholm.

Palme J, Bergmark Å and Bäckman O *et al.* (2002). Welfare trends in Sweden: balancing the books for the 1990s. *Journal of European Social Policy*, **12**, 329–46.

Paoli P and Merllié D (2001). *Third European survey on working conditions 2000*. European Foundation for the Improvement of Living and Working conditions, Dublin.

Putnam RD (1999). *Bowling alone. The collapse and revival of American Community*. Simon and Schuster, New York.

Rahkonen O, Arber S and Lahelma E (1997). Health and social mobility in Britain and Finland. *Scandinavian Journal of Social Medicine*, **25**, 83–92.

Ringbäck W G, Weitoft G, Haglund B, and Rosén M (2000). Mortality among lone mothers in Sweden: a population study. *Lancet*, **355**, 1215–19.

Roos E, Burström B, Saastamoinen P and Lahelma E (2005). A comparative study of the patterning of women's health by family status and employment status in Finland and Sweden. *Social Science and Medicine*, **60**, 2443–51.

Rostgaard T and Lehto J (2001). Health and social care systems: how different is the Nordic model? In: M Kautto, J Fritzell, B Hvinden, J Kvist and H Uusitalo (eds) *Nordic welfare states in the European context*, pp. 137–67. Routledge, London.

Rothstein B and Steinmo S (2002). *Restructuring the welfare state*. Palgrave Macmillan, New York.

Siegrist J (1996). Adverse health effects of high-effort/low-reward conditions. *Journal of Occupational Health Psychology*, **1**, 27–41.

Siegrist J (2000). Place, social exchange and health: proposed sociological framework. *Social Science and Medicine*, **51**, 1283–93.

Silventoinen K and Lahelma E (2002). Health inequalities by education and age in four Nordic countries, 1986 and 1994. *Journal Epidemiology and Community Health*, **56**, 253–8.

Smeeding TM (2002). *Globalization, inequality and the rich countries of the G-20: evidence from the Luxembourg Income Study (LIS)*. LIS Working Paper Series No. 320, Luxembourg.

Stouffer SA, Suchman EA, De Vinney LC, Star A and Williams RM (1949). *The American Soldier*. Princeton University Press, Princeton, NJ.

Swank *et al.* (eds) (2002). *Global capital, political institutions, and policy change in developed welfare states*. Cambridge Studies in Comparative Politics. Cambridge University Press, Cambridge.

Titmuss R (1974). *Social policy*. Allen and Unwin, London.

Vågerö D and Erikson R (1997). Socioeconomic inequalities in morbidity and mortality in Western Europe. *Lancet*, **350**, 516.

Valkonen T (1989). Adult mortality and level of education: a comparison of six countries. In: AJ Fox (ed) *Health inequalities in European countries*, pp. 142–60. Aldershot, Gower.

Valkonen T, Martikainen P, Jalovaara M, Koskinen S, Martelin T and Mäkelä P (2000). Changes in socio-economic inequalities in mortality during an economic boom and recession among middle-aged men and women in Finland. *European Journal of Public Health*, **10**, 274–80.

Warr P (1987). *Work, unemployment and mental health*. Oxford University Press, Oxford.

West P (1991). Rethinking the health selection explanation for health inequalities. *Social Science and Medicine*, **32**, 373–84.

Whitehead M, Burström B and Diderichsen F (2000). Social policies and the pathways to inequalities in health: a comparative analysis of lone mothers in Britain and Sweden. *Social Science and Medicine*, **50**, 255–27.

Wilkinson RG (1996). *Unhealthy societies. The afflictions of inequality*. Routledge, London.

Chapter 10

Socio-economic inequalities in health in Western Europe

From description to explanation to intervention

Johan P. Mackenbach

Introduction

During the last two decades, socio-economic inequalities in health have increasingly been recognized as an important public health issue throughout Western Europe (Anonymous 1997, Mackenbach *et al.* 1997). Reports on socio-economic inequalities in health have appeared in many countries, and the emphasis of academic research has gradually shifted from description to explanation (Davey Smith *et al.* 1994, Vågerö and Illsley 1995, Macintyre 1997). On the basis of a better understanding of the causes of health inequalities, a search for evidence-based strategies to reduce these inequalities has begun (Whitehead and Dahlgren 1991, Dahlgren and Whitehead 1992).

This chapter will review recent European experiences in this area. The chapter begins with a brief overview of the size and pattern of socio-economic inequalities in health in western Europe. It will then review national policy developments, including various innovative approaches and comprehensive blueprints for tackling health inequalities that have been proposed. Finally, it will discuss the types of evidence needed to underpin policies to tackle socio-economic inequalities in health. These requirements will be illustrated with an analysis of some of the new findings on explanation of health inequalities as reported in this volume.

The size and pattern of socio-economic inequalities in health in Western Europe

Mortality

Many western European countries have longitudinal mortality studies in which mortality occurring in the population during a certain period is linked to socio-economic information that was previously collected during a census.

These mortality studies invariably show substantial inequalities in mortality by various indicators of socio-economic status, such as level of education, occupational class, or housing tenure (Kunst *et al.* 1998a, b, Mackenbach *et al.* 1999, Huisman *et al.* 2004). International comparative studies of health inequalities in western Europe have not found systematic differences between countries in the magnitude of inequalities in mortality. Sometimes relatively large or small inequalities in mortality in one country or another have been observed, but these observations were limited to a particular socio-economic indicator (level of education, occupational class, housing tenure), quantitative measure (rate ratio, rate difference), gender and/or age-group, or time-period (Kunst *et al.* 1998a, b, Mackenbach *et al.* 1999, Huisman *et al.* 2004). As an illustration, Figure 10.1 gives an overview of educational differences in total mortality among middle-aged men as observed during the first half of the 1990s in nine European populations. Mortality is between 28 and 53 per cent higher in the lower educational group (primary school or less) than in the higher educational group (secondary school or more). In this particular analysis, relative inequalities are largest in Norway (RR = 1.53, 95 per cent CI: 1.47–1.49), but this is not seen consistently for all socio-economic indicators and outcome measures.

What is evident from this and other analyses is that neither relative nor absolute inequalities in mortality are systematically smaller in the Nordic countries than in other western European countries, as one would expect on the basis of their 'social-democratic' welfare regimes with small income inequalities and low rates of poverty (Mackenbach *et al.* 1997, see Chapter 9 in this volume).

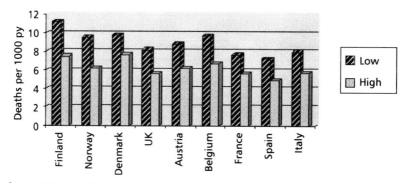

Figure 10.1 Mortality by educational level among men aged 45–59 years, early 1990s, by country.

Note: Italy is represented by the city of Torino and Spain by the region/city of Madrid and Barcelona.

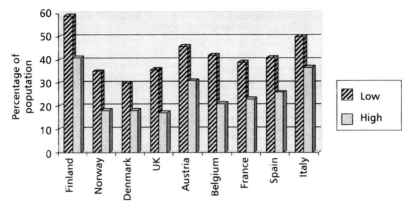

Figure 10.2 Self-assessed health less-than-'good' by educational level among men aged 45–59 years, early 1990s, by country.

Self-reported morbidity

Figure 10.2 presents a similar overview for self-reported morbidity, as measured by the prevalence of less-than-'good' self-assessed health. Inequalities for self-assessed health are substantial in all countries included in this analysis, and the same applies to other forms of self-reported morbidity, such as chronic conditions and long-term disabilities (Cavelaars *et al.* 1998a, b, Huisman *et al.* 2003, Dalstra *et al.* 2005).

When analyses such as those presented in Figure 10.2 are repeated for other socio-economic indicators (occupational class, income level) or other health outcomes (self-reported chronic conditions or disabilities), countries often change position and no systematic patterns have emerged (Cavelaars *et al.* 1998a, b, Huisman *et al.* 2003, Dalstra *et al.* 2005). The only exception is that inequalities in self-assessed health by level of income appear to be smaller in countries with smaller income inequalities (Doorslaer 2000).

Specific diseases

The similarity of relative inequalities in (total) morbidity and mortality across western European populations disappears as soon as we look at specific diseases. For self-reported morbidity such a more detailed analysis is more difficult than for mortality, but recently some encouraging results have been obtained by looking at educational differences in self-reported chronic conditions in a range of western European countries (Dalstra *et al.* 2005).

For mortality, however, disease-specific data are quite robust and show some striking international patterns. The main and consistent finding is of a north-south gradient within Europe, with larger inequalities in cardiovascular disease (particularly ischemic heart disease) mortality in countries like Finland, Norway and the United Kingdom, and smaller inequalities in cardiovascular disease (particularly ischemic heart disease) mortality in countries like France, Spain and Italy (Kunst *et al.* 1998b, Mackenbach *et al.* 2000, Huisman *et al.* 2005). This results in striking differences in the contribution of ischemic heart disease to excess mortality in lower socio-economic groups, as illustrated in Figure 10.3.

It is as if excess total mortality in lower socio-economic groups is made up of compensating contributions of different causes of death: cardiovascular disease in the north, certain cancers (particularly of the gastrointestinal system) and gastrointestinal diseases in the south. Smaller relative inequalities in ischemic heart disease in the south seem to be compensated by larger relative inequalities in cancer mortality, and vice versa in the north. These differences in contribution to excess mortality in lower socio-economic groups mirror differences in cause-of-death pattern for the population as a whole. This suggests that the similarity of relative differences in total mortality is due to the fact that persons with a higher socio-economic status consistently succeed in

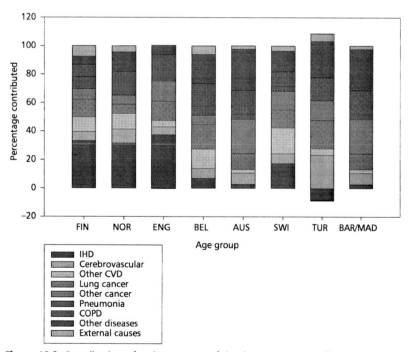

Figure 10.3 Contribution of various causes of death to excess mortality among men in lower educational groups aged 30–74 years, early 1990s, by country.

having a lower mortality level for those diseases that dominate the cause-of-death pattern in their country (Kunst 1997).

Explanations

During the last two decades, research on socio-economic inequalities in health has gradually shifted from description to explanation. Explanatory research has revealed a number of factors and mechanisms that contribute to socio-economic inequalities in health. Examples include unfavourable material living conditions, psychosocial factors, and health-related behaviours that increase the incidence of health problems, and that are more common in the lower socio-economic groups (Davey Smith *et al.* 1994, Vågerö and Illsley 1995, Macintyre 1997, Marmot and Wilkinson 1999, Bartley 2004). Some multivariate analyses have shown that between 40 and 70 per cent of socio-economic inequalities in mortality can be explained from a number of well-known determinants (Marmot *et al.* 1991, Schrijvers *et al.* 1999).

Unfortunately, the availability of comparable data on socio-economic inequalities in specific determinants of mortality and morbidity in a range of western European countries is very limited. The only nationally representative data that can be found in a number of countries are lifestyle-related, such as smoking, fruit and vegetable consumption, and obesity (Cavelaars *et al.* 1997, 2000). As an illustration, Figure 10.4 shows the magnitude of educational inequalities in smoking among middle-aged men in six countries in the early 1990s. These data were collected in national health interviews or multi-purpose surveys, and results on educational inequalities resemble those obtained with data collected in Eurobarometer surveys or in the European Community Household Panel. Relative inequalities in smoking differ considerably between countries, with considerable consistency between different socio-economic indicators (level of education, occupational class,

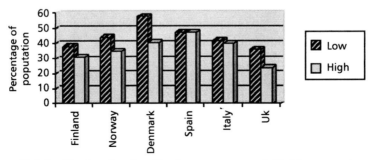

Figure 10.4 Smoking by educational level among men aged 45–59 years, early 1990s, by country.

level of income). Larger inequalities are found in Finland, Norway, Denmark and the UK. Italy and Spain have very small inequalities in smoking among middle-aged men, while among middle-aged women in these countries an inverse pattern of inequalities in smoking has been observed, with lower educated women smoking less than higher educated women (Cavelaars *et al.* 1997, 2000, Huisman *et al.* (in press)).

This north-south gradient in social patterning of smoking corresponds with the north-south gradient in inequalities in ischemic heart disease mortality described above. More generally, variations between countries in lifetime histories of smoking by socio-economic group, as reflected in lung cancer death rates, may explain a considerable part of variations between countries in total mortality by socio-economic group (Mackenbach *et al.* 2004). This should not distract from the fact that the social patterning of smoking is in itself determined by many other factors, e.g. material living conditions and psychosocial factors, and that other factors also contribute substantially and directly to inequalities in health (Lynch *et al.* 1997, Droomers *et al.* 2002). But it is quite obvious that smoking presents an important target for policies to tackle health inequalities, at least in the west and north of Europe.

Policy developments vis-à-vis health inequalities in Western Europe

National policy developments

Different countries are in widely different phases of awareness of, and willing-ness to take action on, socio-economic inequalities in health. Figure 10.5 illus-trates these differences for nine countries from various parts of Europe (Mackenbach *et al.* 2003a). Four common milestones in policy development have been distinguished: high-profile independent reports recommending research or policy on health inequalities; national research programs on health inequalities; government advisory committees recommending policies to reduce health inequalities; and coordinated government action to reduce health inequalities.

The first event included in Figure 10.5 is the publication of the Black report in 1980 in Britain (Townsend and Davidson 1992) – an event which has spurred research in Britain and increased awareness of health inequalities in the rest of Europe. It took more than a decade before further action was taken in Britain, first in the form of national research programmes and important government and non-government reports (Department of Health 1995), then culminating in the Independent Inquiry published in 1998 (Acheson 1998a). National governments in several other countries responded earlier, probably because

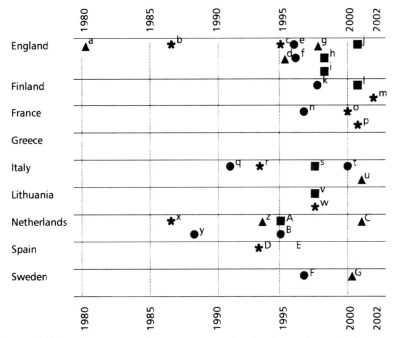

Figure 10.5 Timelines representing concurrent policy developments in nine European countries.

* High-profile independent report recommending policy action on health inequalities

• Start of national research programme on health inequalities

▲ Report of government advisory commission focusing on health inequalities reduction

■ Government policy document focusing on health inequalities reduction

a Black Report 1980

b Health Divide 1987

c Tackling Inequalities in Health; an Agenda for Action; King's Fund 1995

d Variations in health: What can the Department of Health and the NHS do?; Department of Health, 1995

e Economic and Social Research Council's Health Variations Program 1996–2001

f Department of Health's Health Inequalities Research and Development initiative 1996–1999

g Independent Inquiry into Inequalities in Health Report; D. Acheson 1998

h Department of Health. Saving lives: our healthier nation. London, Stationery Office 1999

i Department of Health. Reducing health inequalities: an action report. London, Stationery Office 1999.

j Department of Health. From vision to reality. London, Stationery Office 2001

k Health and Other Welfare Differences between Population Groups 1998–2000, Academy of Finland, 1998

l Government Resolution on the Health 2015 public health programma, Ministry of Social Affairs and Health 2001

m Kohti terveyden tasa-arvoa (Towards equality in health), Kangas I, Keskimäki I, Koskinen S, Manderbacka K, Lahelma E, Prättälä R, Sihto M (eds), 2002

n INSERM (National Health Research Institute) Research Program 1997

Figure 10.5 *(Continued)*

[o] Les inégalités sociales de santé (Inequalities in Health); Leclerc *et al.* 2000

[p] Précarisation, risques et santé (Precariousness, Risks and Health); Joubert *et al.* 2001

[q] Health Department and the Piedmont Region national research program 1991

[r] L'equità nella salute in Italia. Rapporto sulle diseguaglianze in sanità (Equity in Health in Italy. Report on Social Inequalities In Health); Costa and Faggiano 1994

[s] Piano Sanitario Nazionale 1998–2000. Un patto di solidarietà per la salute (National Health Plan 1998–2000). A Solidarity Agreement for Health 1998

[t] National Research Program 2000–2002

[u] Orientamenti bioetici per l'equita nella salute (Bioethical guidelines for equity in health), National Committee for Bioethics 2001

[v] Lithuanian Health Program 1997–2010; Ministry of Health 1998

[w] Equity in health and healthcare in Lithuania. A situation analysis; WHO/ Swedish International Development Agency 1998

[x] De ongelijke verdeling van gezondheid (The Differential Distribution of Health); Scientific Council for Governmental Policy 1987

[y] First National Research Program 1989–1993

[z] Programmacommissie Sociaal-economische gezondheidsverschillen. Onderzoeksprogramma sociaal-economische gezondheidsverschillen; eindverslag en aanbevelingen. Rijswijk: Ministerie van WVC, 1994.

[A] Health and Wellbeing; Ministry of Public Health, Welfare and Sport 1995

[B] Second National Research Program 1995–2001

[C] Sociaal-economische gezondheidsverschillen verkleinen. Eindrapportage en beleidsaanbevelingen van de Programmacommissie SEGV-II (Reducing Socioeconomic Inequalities in Health. Final Report and Policy Recommendations of the Program Committee SEIH-II) 2001

[D] Diferencias y desigualdades en salud en España (Differences and inequalities in Health in Spain); Regidor *et al.*, 1994

[E] Desigualdades sociales en salud en España (Social Inequalities in Health in Spain); Navarro and Benach 1996

[F] Program of Health Inequalities Research; Social Research Council, the Medical Research Council and the National Institute of Public Health 1997

[G] Ministry of Health and Social Affairs. Hälsa på lika villkor – nationella mål för folkhälsan. Slutbetänkande av nationella folkhälsokommittén (Health on equal terms – final proposal on national targets for public health). Stockholm: Ministry of Health and Social Affairs 2000. (SOU 2000:91)

Source: Mackenbach JP *et al.* 2003a (Reprinted from *The Lancet*, Vol. 362, Mackenbach JP, Bakker MJ, Tackling socioeconomic inequalities in health: analysis of European experiences, pp. 1409–14, 2003, with permission from Elsevier.)

of differences in political climate. In the Netherlands (late 1980s) (Programmacommissie Sociaal-economischvgezondheidsverschillen 1994) and Italy (early 1990s) (Costa *et al.* 2002), heightened awareness of health inequalities, partly generated by the Black report, led to government-sponsored research programmes in this field. In Finland (mid-1980s) (Ministry of Social Affairs and Health, Helsinki 1986) and Sweden (early 1990s) (Ministry of Health and Social Affairs, Stockholm 1991), inequalities in health were addressed in major government policy documents on public health generally (not shown in Figure 10.5).

Whitehead has proposed a schematic 'action spectrum' to characterize the stage of diffusion of ideas on socio-economic inequalities in health (Whitehead 1998). Starting with a primordial stage in which socio-economic inequalities in health are not even measured, the spectrum covers the stages of 'measurement', 'recognition', 'awareness', 'denial/indifference', 'concern', 'will to take action', 'isolated initiatives', 'more structured developments' and 'comprehensive coordinated policy'. Among the countries included in our analysis, which was carried out in 2002, Greece is the only one that finds itself still in a pre-measurement stage. Data on socio-economic inequalities in health are almost completely lacking, and awareness of the issue is limited to a small number of academics who do not have structural research funding for studies in this area (Tountas 2002). Spain, after a period with heightened awareness due to the publication of a Spanish 'Black Report' (Navarro *et al.* 1996), currently finds itself in a 'denial/indifference' stage, largely because of a change in political colour of the national government. France and Italy both are in a 'concern' stage: important reports on socio-economic inequalities in health have been published (Leclerc *et al.* 2000, Chauvin and Lebas 1998, Costa and Faggiano 1994), and policy-makers are increasingly paying attention to the issue. Lithuania, after the fall of the Soviet empire, has rapidly reached a 'will to take action' stage, as evidenced by parliamentary resolutions and reports from government advisory councils (Grabauskas *et al.* 2002). The Netherlands and Sweden are in a 'more structured developments' stage, with national research programmes as well as high-level advisory committees that have recently issued comprehensive policy advice on how to reduce socio-economic inequalities in health (Programmacommissie Sociaal-Economische GezondheidsVerschillen-tweede fase 2001, Ministry of Health and Social Affairs 1986).

The international comparison suggests that Britain, after a period of lagging behind other European countries, is now ahead of continental Europe in developing and implementing policies to reduce socio-economic inequalities in health. It is the only country where policy advice has led to a significant number of new government initiatives specifically addressing health inequalities. Since the introduction of devolution in 1999 there have been a growing number of differences in health and other public policies between different parts of the United Kingdom, and it has therefore become difficult to make general statements. Our analysis has focused on England, and this seems to have entered a 'comprehensive coordinated policy' stage. Many recommendations from the Independent Inquiry have been accepted by the government in major policy documents (Department of Health 1999a, 1999b, 2001, 2004), and a series of new policies have been implemented ranging from neighbourhood renewal programmes to a fuel poverty strategy and from a national school fruit scheme to a child tax credit. Although from a European perspective some of these policies could be seen as a form of catching up (similar programmes were adopted long ago in other countries), the level of official government commitment is certainly unique at this time.

Innovative approaches

During our inventory of national policy developments and an additional policy area-specific literature search we identified a number of specific innovative approaches to reduce health inequalities (Mackenbach and Bakker 2002). Documentation on the development, implementation and evaluation of these innovations was collected, and we classified them in five main areas: policy steering mechanisms, labour market and working conditions, consumption and health-related behaviour, health care, and territorial approaches. Table 10.1 lists examples in each of these categories. For each of the innovations (with the exception of policy steering mechanisms) there is at least some empirical evidence suggesting that they can help to reduce health inequalities. A full discussion of these innovative approaches can be found elsewhere (Mackenbach and Bakker 2002). Here we will only highlight a few examples in the areas of 'labour market and working conditions', 'health-related behaviour', and 'health care'.

Health inequalities are partly due to labour market and working conditions. Swedish labour market policies enforce strong employment protection and active promotion of labour market participation for citizens with chronic illness. A comparison with England suggests that these policies have been effective in protecting vulnerable groups from labour market exclusion during the recession of the 1990s (Burström *et al.* 2000). In France, occupational health services are mandatory and include an annual health check for every employee. This provides a good setting for introducing preventive activities for those who otherwise have few medical contacts, particularly those in manual occupations. Randomized controlled trials within this setting have shown that interventions aimed at detection and treatment of hypertension and smoking cessation were successful (Lang *et al.* 1995, 2000). In Italy, a financial crisis in the early 1990s led to a reform of the pension scheme and a postponement of retirement age. Trade unions called attention to socio-economic inequalities in life expectancy, and negotiated a one-year reduction in retirement age for manual workers (Costa *et al.* 2002). Improvements of working conditions have made important contributions to reducing health inequalities in the past, but a lot remains to be done. In the Netherlands a recent intervention study suggests that task rotation among garbage collectors

Table 10.1 Innovative approaches for tackling socio-economic inequalities in health developed during the 1990s in various European countries.

Policy steering mechanisms
  Quantitative policy targets
    Reduction of inequalities in 11 intermediate outcomes (poverty, smoking, working conditions. . . .) – Netherlands
  Health inequalities impact assessment
    Qualitative assessment of impact on health inequalities of EC agricultural policy – Sweden

Labour market and working conditions
  Universal approaches
    Strong employment protection and active labour market policies for chronically ill citizens – Sweden
    Occupational health services offering annual check-ups and preventive interventions to all employees – France
  Targeted approaches
    Reduction in retirement age for manual workers – Italy
    Job rotation among dustmen – Netherlands

Health-related behaviours
  Universal approaches
    Serve low-fat food products through mass catering in schools and workplaces – Finland
  Targeted approaches
    Multi-method intervention to reduce smoking among low income women – Britain

Health care
  Improving quality of care
    Nurse practitioners to support GPs working in deprived areas – Netherlands
  Working with other agencies
    Community strategies led by local government agencies, but integrating care across all the local public sector services, including health – England

Territorial approaches
  Comprehensive health strategies for deprived areas
    Health Action Zones – England
    Municipal health policy towards Ciutat Vella, Barcelona – Spain

Source: Mackenbach JP *et al.* 2003a. (Reprinted from *The Lancet*, Vol. 362, Mackenbach JP, Bakker MJ, Tackling socio-economic inequalities in health: analysis of European experiences, pp. 1409–14, 2003, with permission from Elsevier.)

reduces sickness absenteeism. Rotation of tasks (truck driving and minicontainer loading) reduces physical load and possibly also increases job control (Kuijer *et al.* 1999).

Health-related behaviours like food consumption, smoking and physical exercise also contribute to socio-economic inequalities in health. Finnish nutrition policies have followed the Nordic welfare ideology where universalism has been the general principle. School children, students and employees in Finland receive free or subsidized meals at school or workplace, and special dietary guidelines have been implemented ensuring the use of low-fat food products. This has probably contributed to the favourable trend of narrowing socio-economic inequalities in use of butter and high-fat milk in Finland (Prättälä *et al.* 1992). In many countries, smoking is increasingly concentrated in lower socio-economic groups, and reviews show that a variety of policies and interventions is effective in reducing smoking in these groups. Whereas the price weapon (raising excise taxes) is very effective, its regressive impact on the poorest smokers who cannot stop should be counteracted by active promotion of the use of nicotine replacement therapy and other cessation support. Low income women are a group where it is particularly difficult to change smoking behaviour, and a promising Scottish initiative therefore combined various approaches (community development, drama and poetry, fitness, cessation services, social support) (Gaunt-Richardson *et al.* 1999).

Universal access to effective health care, regardless of income or other forms of social disadvantage, is another important factor. Unequal access to health care services (according to need) may aggravate socio-economic inequalities in health or even cause them. In addition, health care can contribute to reducing health inequalities by offering dedicated services to lower socio-economic groups and by taking the lead in working with other agencies. In the Netherlands, nurse practitioners have been introduced in general practice, and an intervention study in practices operating in deprived areas suggests that counselling of congestive obstructive pulmonary disease/asthma patients resulted in better compliance with therapy and reduced complications (Sorgdrager *et al.* 2001). In England, recent health service reforms gave local health authorities the lead responsibility for working with other agencies to improve health and reduce inequalities. The key integrating device is the production of a three-year rolling plan for health, which feeds into a wider community strategy, committing all the local public sector services to a programme to improve the economic, social and environmental well-being of each area (Department of Health 2001).

Blueprints for comprehensive strategies

As it is unlikely that any single policy or intervention will significantly reduce socio-economic inequalities in health, packages of policies and interventions of a more comprehensive nature have been devised by government advisory committees in Britain, Sweden and the Netherlands (Table 10.2).

Table 10.2 Comparison of three blueprints for comprehensive packages of policies and interventions to reduce inequalities in health

British Independent Inquiry into inequalities in health (1998)

39 main recommendations (123 with sub-clauses)

Seven overarching policy areas reviewed, corresponding to the major departments of state:

- Taxation and social security
- Education
- Employment
- Housing and environment
- Mobility, transport and pollution
- Nutrition and the common agricultural policy
- National Health Service

Demographic factors over the life course considered, including

- Mothers, children and families
- Young people and adults of working age
- Older people
- Ethnicity
- Gender

Three priority areas are emphasized as crucial to addressing inequalities

1. Health inequalities impact assessment
2. A high priority for the health of families with children
3. Reduction in income inequalities and improvement of living standards of poor households

The Dutch programme committee on socioeconomic inequalities in health (2001)

26 recommendations

Four specific strategies:

1. Reduction of inequalities in education, income and other socio-economic factors
   e.g. no increase in income inequalities; anti-poverty measures; benefits to counter health effects of poverty
2. Reduction of the negative effects of health problems on socio-economic position
   e.g. decent benefits for work-incapacity; improved labour market participation of chronically ill
3. Reduction of the negative effects of socio-economic position on health
   e.g. reduction of smoking, overweight, physical and psychosocial work load in lower se-groups
4. Improve access and quality of healthcare for lower socio-economic groups
   e.g. preserve equal access; strengthen primary care in deprived neighbourhoods

Eleven quantitative targets relating to intermediate outcomes.

In general, strong emphasis on continuation of research, development, monitoring and evaluation.

Swedish National Public Health Commission (2000)

18 health policy objectives

Six overarching themes:

1. Strengthening social capital
   e.g. reduce poverty; reduce segregation in housing; reduced isolation and loneliness
2. Growing up in a satisfactory environment
   e.g. secure parent-child bond; schools that strengthen pupils' self-confidence

Table 10.2 *(continued)*

   3. Improving conditions at work
      e.g. low unemployment; adapt physical and mental work demands;
      reduced overtime
   4. Creating a satisfactory physical environment
      e.g. green areas and playgrounds; high standards of building; safe traffic
      environment
   5. Stimulating health-promoting life habits
      e.g. more physical exercise; reduce overweight; reduce unwanted pregnancies
   6. Developing a satisfactory infrastructure for health
      e.g. strengthening prevention; coordination of public health efforts;
      intensified research
Development of 'indicators for achievement' recommended.

Source: Mackenbach JP *et al*. 2003a. (Reprinted from *The Lancet*, Vol. 362, Mackenbach JP, Bakker MJ, Tackling socio-economic inequalities in health: analysis of European experiences, pp. 1409–14, 2003, with permission from Elsevier.)

The Black Report, mentioned above, contained the first example of such a comprehensive strategy (Townsend and Davidson 1992) but was received coolly and largely ignored by the Conservative government that was in power when it was issued in 1980. Further high-profile reports, such as The Health Divide (Whitehead 1992), stimulated widespread debate in the late 1980s, but were rejected by the government of the day. By the mid-1990s, however, the political climate had softened, and the King's Fund revisited the area and made a systematic attempt to review the scientific evidence for effective policies and interventions to reduce socio-economic inequalities in health (Benzeval *et al*. 1995). The King's Fund report paved the way for the Independent Inquiry into Inequalities in Health, held by the Acheson Committee. The committee came up with 39 recommendations (123 in total, counting sub-clauses) (Acheson 1998a). Without a doubt this is the most comprehensive set of recommendations ever prepared. It has consequently been criticized for its lack of clear priorities (Davey Smith *et al*. 1998), although three areas were singled out as priorities in the report (Acheson 1998b), as detailed in Table 10.2. There is a certain emphasis on addressing 'upstream' factors like income, education and employment, while recommendations on 'downstream' factors, like health-related behaviour, are presented as part of more general strategies directed towards groups defined in terms of age, gender and ethnicity. The role of the National Health Service in reducing health inequalities is presented under a separate heading, probably to emphasize that even though deficiencies in health services are not a major cause of inequalities in health status, the health sector has an important part to play in any strategy to address observed health inequalities. Since the publication of the report, important progress has been made in implementing a number of its recommendations (Department of Health 1999a, b, 2001, 2004).

Two recent reports from the Netherlands and Sweden provide an interesting contrast. In the Netherlands a national Program Committee on Socio-economic Inequalities in Health has recently issued a set of 26 specific recommendations (Programmacommissie Sociaal-Economische GezondheidsVerschillen-tweede fase 2001, Mackenbach and Stronks 2002, 2004). The committee is commonly called after its chairman, Albeda, a former Christian-Democrat Minister of Social Affairs. The committee had an equal representation of scientists and policy-makers, the latter representing different political parties. The recommendations were partly based on a series of intervention studies in which 12 different interventions addressing inequalities in health were subjected to, mostly quasi-experimental, process or outcome evaluations. A consultation exercise involving policy-makers and practitioners in various fields was part of the exercise (Stronks and Hulshof 2001). The recommendations were grouped in four strategies to address four different entry-points: reduction of inequalities in socio-economic factors; reduction of the negative effect of health on socio-economic position; reduction of the negative effect of socio-economic disadvantage on health (through reduced exposure to specific risk factors); and improved access and quality of health care. These entry-points were derived from a simple and pragmatic model that was devised to help policy-makers understand how socio-economic inequalities in health are generated. Examples of recommendations include 'no further increase in income inequality', 'no cuts in disability benefits', 'increase labour participation of the chronically ill', 'reduce physically demanding work', 'increase tobacco taxation', 'implement school health policies' and 'strengthen primary care in deprived areas' (Programmacommissie Sociaal-Economische GezondheidsVerschillen-tweede fase 2001, Mackenbach and Stronks 2002). Due to recent political instabilities in the Netherlands, the national government has only recently started to implement some of the recommendations of the Albeda committee. At the local and regional level, however, many new initiatives have been taken to tackle health inequalities (Mackenbach and Stronks 2004).

In Sweden the National Public Health Commission, a committee consisting of representatives of all political parties, scientific experts and advisers from governmental and non-governmental organizations, has recently developed a new national health policy with a strong focus on reducing health inequalities. The commission used a conceptual model resembling the Dutch model, but with contextual factors and the social consequences of disease added. Although the exercise involved a review of scientific evidence, like in the Independent

Inquiry this review focused on explanations of inequalities in health, not on the evaluation of policies and interventions. It further involved extensive consultation of numerous organizations, and the proposal itself includes action by a wide range of actors in society. The commission formulated 18 health policy objectives grouped in six large areas: strengthening social capital; growing up in a satisfactory environment; improving conditions at work; creating a satisfactory physical environment; stimulating health-promoting life habits; and developing a satisfactory infrastructure for health. Specific factors addressed by the strategy range from contextual factors such as social cohesion and housing segregation (with effects on children's educational opportunities) to work organization (with effects on job strain) and tobacco and alcohol consumption. The commission recommended development of quantitative targets related to each of these policy objectives, but although specific targets were presented in draft versions of the strategy, these were withdrawn as the process progressed (Ministry of Health and Social Affairs, Stockholm 2000).

Towards evidence-based policy-making to tackle socio-economic inequalities in health

The evidence base for current policies to tackle health inequalities

Within western Europe, there is considerable diversity in the way scientific evidence has been used to underpin policies to reduce health inequalities. This is illustrated by the way the three comprehensive blueprints mentioned above were developed. The Acheson Committee commissioned 18 reviews of the evidence covering seven overarching policy areas, together with major sociodemographic factors over the life course. Much of the evidence in the commissioned reviews related to the contribution of specific factors to the explanation of health inequalities, not to the effectiveness of policies and interventions tackling them (Macintyre *et al.* 2001). By contrast, the Dutch strategy was developed at the end of a six-year research programme in which 12 studies were carried out to assess the effectiveness of various intervention options. The results of these studies were then discussed with experts and policy-makers, to see how these fitted into the existing evidence-base and in current policy (Stronks and Hulshof 2001). Although the approach proved only partly successful, because some entry-points for policy were not covered by evaluation studies, and some evaluation studies failed while others had design weaknesses, in the end a sizeable fraction of policy recommendations was related to specific results of the programme (Mackenbach and Stronks

2002). In the Swedish case the emphasis again was strongly on evidence relating to the explanation of health inequalities. The process was one of consultation with practitioners and policy-makers that ensured their commitment with the final recommendations. Evidence demonstrating that the strategies will actually work in terms of reducing health inequalities was not provided (Ministry of Health and Social Affairs, Stockholm 2000).

This diversity is also seen in the opinions of different researchers on what type of evidence is needed to underpin policies and interventions in this field. There are those who argue that in view of the urgency of starting to tackle health inequalities ('doing nothing is not an option') (Petticrew *et al.* 2004), one should be prepared to start intervening on the basis of plausibility. Political windows of opportunity are usually short, e.g. four years at most, and they may be closed before careful evaluation studies have been conducted (Whitehead *et al.* 2004). A parallel has been drawn with nineteenth-century public health interventions for which controlled intervention studies have never been done, but which were implemented on the basis of plausibility and have proven to be highly successful (Davey Smith *et al.* 2001). Under the pressure of politicians wanting to see rapid results, the best that can be achieved in terms of scientific evaluation may then be large-scale implementation accompanied by a real time evaluation study of the intervention, concurrent with its implementation, using some quasi-experimental design (before-after study, interrupted time-series study, etc.) (Macintyre 2003).

On the other hand, there are those who argue that this is a strategy with serious risks. Like in other areas of social and health policy, the actual results of policies and interventions to reduce health inequalities could easily be counterintuitive. There are many historical examples of 'plausible' interventions and policies that did not work, or actually had adverse effects (Macintyre *et al.* 2001). The fact that there are no systematic differences between countries in the magnitude of health inequalities, despite large differences in health, social and economic policies, should also warn us against optimism about the effects of policies and interventions that seem plausible. Shouldn't one expect the magnitude of health inequalities in the Nordic countries, with their long histories of egalitarian economic, social, and health care policies, to be smaller than in other western European countries? The fact that this is not the case, suggests that policies which could plausibly be seen as conducive to reducing health inequalities, may actually not be of much help, or at the very least far from sufficient. Several explanations have been suggested, including that the generous 'welfare state regimes' in the Nordic countries may actually have enabled people in lower socio-economic groups to participate in an affluent life-style, including smoking, lack of physical exercise, overeating, and excessive alcohol consumption (Chapter 9 in this volume). In addition to that, one could argue that any investment in reducing health inequalities should be justified on the basis of a comparison of its cost-effectiveness with that of other possible investments in health and well-being, and that producing credible evidence is therefore essential (Oliver 2001). Pleas have been made for more systematically collecting evidence on the (cost-) effectiveness of inter- ventions and policies to reduce health inequalities (Macintyre *et al.* 2001).

What types and levels of evidence are needed?

Despite the disagreements on what types and levels of evidence are needed before policies and interventions to reduce health inequalities are implemented, there is a general consensus that collection of such evidence is needed. The next question then is what types and levels of evidence should be collected. Schematically, the evidence-base underpinning decisions to implement a policy or intervention to tackle health inequalities could be built up in the following sequence:

◆ Creating a theoretical rationale for the intervention or policy: identifying factors which make a substantial, independent contribution to the expla- nation of health inequalities.

◆ Developing an intervention or policy which could target these factors: adapting existing, or creating new, interventions or policies which are likely to do more good than harm, which will differentially benefit lower socio- economic groups, and which can be implemented on a sufficiently large scale to have an impact on health inequalities at the population level.

◆ Demonstrating the (cost-)effectiveness of this intervention or policy: showing empirically that the policy or intervention reduces health inequal- ities in settings similar to that in which it will be implemented, taking into account any harmful side-effects, and to an extent that justifies its cost.

For the first step, one must rely on evidence from carefully designed observa- tional studies, such as longitudinal (or prospective cohort) studies in which exposure to low socio-economic status and specific health determinants has been measured at baseline, and health outcomes are measured during follow- up. A number of such longitudinal studies have been set up over the past decades in some Western European countries, and have contributed impor- tantly to the evidence base (Marmot *et al.* 1991, Mackenbach *et al.* 1994, Ford *et al.* 1994, Website). A variety of factors has been shown to make important contributions to the explanation of health inequalities, particularly inequal- ities in mortality or incidence of cardiovascular disease. Evidence on other outcomes is much more scarce. Because of the complexity of the explanation of health inequalities, in which chains of interconnected factors are thought to be operating over the life-course, one must be careful in interpreting the results of these studies. It is not necessarily the case that factors which have been identified by conventionally designed cohort studies, indeed make an 'independent' contribution to the explanation of health inequalities, in the sense that if this particular factor would be removed, the magnitude of health inequalities can be assumed to be reduced by its contribution as measured in multivariate analyses. Grading systems for assessing the quality of evidence from observational studies have not yet been developed, but are being developed now (Elm and Egger 2004). Preferably, development of policies or interventions should be based on systematic reviews of such evidence which take differences in the quality of separate studies into account. It is important to be aware of the fact that the explanation of health inequalities, in terms of specific 'downstream' factors, is likely to be substantially different between western European countries, and that theoretical rationales constructed for one country may have limited generalizability to other countries. This was illustrated above with the example of smoking.

Generally speaking, it is unlikely that suitable policies or interventions which effectively target factors identified in the first step are already available. Many of the factors known to be involved in the explanation of health inequalities, such as working and housing conditions, health-related behaviours, or psychosocial stressors, have been known to be health determinants for a long time, and many of them have been addressed by health or intersectoral policies. The fact that they still make important contributions to the explanation of health inequalities implies that current policies to address these factors are insufficiently effective in lower socio-economic groups. More powerful and/or tailored approaches will therefore have to be developed, and carefully assessed, e.g. with regard to the balance between benefits and harms. In this stage of development, powerful evaluation designs are usually not necessary, just as in the case of drugs development where so-called phase I and II studies are usually small and uncontrolled (Thomson *et al.* 2004). Because of the scale of the problem of health inequalities, which requires changing the gradient of health problems in whole populations, it is crucial that policies and interventions are developed which can effectively reach large sections of the population.

After the development stage, 'promising' new approaches will need to be evaluated for their effectiveness under real-life circumstances. Clearly, randomized controlled trials will not always be feasible, particularly for the evaluation of policies and interventions that are applied on a population-wide scale. Sometimes, Community Intervention Trials, in which groups of people (school classes, neighbourhoods, . . .) instead of individuals are allocated to the intervention and control condition, will then be a good alternative. But in many circumstances one will have to rely on quasi-experimental or even observational designs to inform policy-makers on the effectiveness of new approaches. Controlled before-after studies or interrupted time-series designs could then be used, or observational studies of 'natural experiments', e.g. by making comparisons between countries (Thomson *et al.* 2004). Systems for grading the quality of evidence from experimental studies have been available for some time already, but recently new grading systems which can also be used for grading evidence from non-experimental studies have been developed (Eccles *et al.* 2003), as well as a comprehensive grading system ('GRADE'), which integrates a number of different aspects relating to the quality of evidence and strength of recommendations across a wide range of interventions and contexts (GRADE Working Group 2004). For each important outcome, the latter approach recommends performing a systematic review of evaluation studies, and assessing four key elements: study design, study quality, consistency across studies, and 'directness' (an aggregate of various aspects covering external validity, surrogate versus final outcomes, etc.). It also recommends looking explicitly at the balance of benefits and harms, and the balance of net benefits and costs.

A complicating factor in evaluating the effectiveness of policies and interventions to reduce health inequalities is that this effectiveness should be measured in terms of favourably changing the distribution of health problems in the population, not of reducing the rate of health problems in a particular group. A full study design therefore requires the measurement, in one or more experimental populations and one or more control populations, of changes over time in the magnitude of health inequalities. Any other design, such as an experimental study of changes over time in the rate of health problems in lower socio-economic groups only, requires rather strong assumptions to be made, in this case on the absence of health effects in higher socio-economic groups (Mackenbach and Gunning-Schepers 1997). Fulfilling this requirement is rather difficult in experimental study designs, which is an additional argument for accepting quasi-experimental and observational evidence in this area.

Results of the ESF programme: new insights for policy?

The studies performed in the framework of the ESF programme on 'Social variations in health expectancy', and reported in various chapters of this volume, have substantially strengthened the evidence base for policies to reduce health inequalities. Also, by bringing together researchers and research findings from different western European (and North American) countries, generalizability of findings beyond a single national context has been promoted. In terms of the three steps outlined above, these studies have contributed to creating and strengthening theoretical rationales for policies and interventions to reduce health inequalities. By providing new, and strengthening old, evidence for the explanation of health inequalities, these studies have helped to shape future policies and interventions. To illustrate how this might be the case, I will briefly discuss two examples.

The ESF Working Group on Life-course approaches has brought together evidence from a number of western European countries confirming and further elaborating previous research findings, which suggest that childhood socio-economic disadvantage makes an independent and substantial contribution to explaining inequalities in adult ill-health (see Chapter 2 in this volume). It is difficult to imagine that a formal systematic review (which has not yet been done for this particular study question) will not confirm this conclusion. Many studies have also pointed to specific factors which may be involved in the connection between childhood socio-economic disadvantage and adult ill-health (childhood health problems, behavioural problems, educational attainment etc.), and the theoretical rationale for policies and interventions targeting these factors is therefore relatively well developed. The main problem is that such policies and interventions will probably only result in substantial reductions in health inequalities after several decades have elapsed – and that they therefore cannot be seen as a solution for current problems.

This is also an area in which many different policies and interventions have already been developed and evaluated, at least with regard to their effects in the population as a whole or in specific subgroups. A recent review has shown that there is reasonably good evidence for the effectiveness of a variety of policies and interventions targeting specific factors that may be involved in the connection between childhood socio-economic disadvantage and adult ill-health, particularly physical and mental health problems and health-related behaviours in children and adolescents (Mielck *et al.* 2002). Also, there is some evidence that social and educational interventions may be effective in reducing some of the disadvantage of children from lower socio-economic background (HM Treasury 1998). Therefore, it is likely that a combination of policies and interventions can be made which can have a substantial impact on adult health inequalities in the future.

The next step then is to evaluate such a package. Some first steps in this direction have recently been made in the UK, with the implementation and evaluation of the Sure Start programme, an early-childhood programme designed to promote the development of children aged 0 to 3 in disadvantaged areas. The services include childcare, primary health care, early education and income support for families. An independent evaluation including potential health effects has been planned (Roberts 2000). Long-term follow-up will be needed to see whether health inequalities at later ages are reduced. Developing and implementing more such packages, and evaluating them as to their (cost-)effectiveness in reducing health inequalities, should be recommended to policy-makers around western Europe, because this is essential for further building up the evidence base.

The ESF Working Group on Psychosocial stress, work and health has brought together evidence from a number of western European countries confirming and further elaborating previous research findings, which suggest that psychosocial factors and their biological responses, such as psychosocial stressors, biological stress markers, coping, and low control beliefs mediate socio-economic inequalities in adult ill-health (see chapters 5, 6, and 7 in this volume). This is an exciting research area at the frontier of current knowledge, which is likely to have scientific paybacks extending far beyond the field of socio-economic inequalities in health. While there still is controversy about the independent contributions that these factors make to the explanation of health inequalities (Lynch *et al.* 2000), the time seems to have to come to start thinking about the development of policies and interventions that could effectively influence these factors at the scale required for reducing health inequalities at the population level.

Research and development underpinning this next step is still very much in its infancy. Treatments or preventive measures that address psychosocial stressors or their biological responses (such as stress management or pharmacological methods) will not necessarily be valuable in a public health context (see chapter 5 in this volume). There are some examples of studies suggesting positive effects of empowerment strategies, but such effects are far from well-established (Wallerstein 2002). It is likely that in order to be effective, policies and interventions will not only have to address the psychosocial factors, but also their environmental determinants, e.g. by increasing actual control and power for individuals with a lower socio-economic status (Syme 1989) (see Chapter 4 in this volume). Some evidence that increasing control in the workplace may be effective in reducing health problems has already been collected (Bond and Bunce 2001). Policy-makers should be advised to support the development and small-scale implementation and evaluation of policies and interventions which are likely to do more good than harm, and which will differentially benefit lower socio-economic groups. The emphasis should be on policies and interventions which can potentially be implemented on a sufficiently large scale to have an impact on health inequalities at the population level. If this development stage proves successful, and results in packages of policies and interventions which could really have an impact, cost-effectiveness will have to be determined using appropriate research designs.

Conclusions

Whether it will actually be possible to substantially reduce socio-economic inequalities in health remains an open question. Western European trends in inequalities in mortality during the last decades of the twentieth century have generally shown a widening of the gap in relative terms, and at best a stable situation in absolute terms (Mackenbach *et al.* 2003b). This was despite the WHO equity target for the period 1985–2000 (WHO 1985), but as previous analyses have shown, despite good intentions in some countries, scale and intensity of efforts aiming to reduce health inequalities have been very modest, at least until 1998 (Mackenbach *et al.* 2003a). The analysis reported in this chapter shows that it was only towards the end of the 1990s that a few countries reached a stage of policy development in which serious efforts can be, and sometimes are, considered.

There is a lot of good news too, however. First, in western Europe during the 1990s there has been enormous progress in explanatory research, and this has identified a large number of targets for policies and interventions to tackle health inequalities. The ESF programme has made an important contribution to this effort, mainly by further strengthening the theoretical rationale for these policies and interventions. Second, there has also been a beginning of research and development for effective interventions and policies to tackle health inequalities. While this is still a modest beginning, it does put us in a better position to reduce socio-economic inequalities in health in the coming decades. A number of innovative approaches have been developed for which there is at least some evidence of effectiveness. Blueprints of comprehensive packages have been developed in several countries that have a sound theoretical basis and clear inspirational value, and that have been taken or are being taken seriously by policy-makers. Progress in research and increased awareness among policy-makers have created an enormous 'window of opportunity' that should be used for moving policy forward.

Developing effective strategies to reduce health inequalities is a daunting task. No single country has the capacity to contribute more than a fraction of the necessary knowledge. This is a matter not only of restricted manpower or financial resources for research, but also of restricted opportunities for implementing and evaluating policies and interventions. Some policies can be implemented and evaluated in some countries and not in others, either because they have already been implemented or because they are politically infeasible. International exchange is therefore necessary to increase learning speed. As this chapter illustrates, such international exchange is feasible and informative, and should be supported strongly by international agencies such as the European Union.

References

Acheson D (1998a). *Independent inquiry into inequalities in health report*. The Stationery Office, London.

Acheson D (1998b). Report on inequalities in health did give priority for steps to be tackled. (letter). *British Medical Journal*, **317**, 1659.

Anonymous (1997). Health inequality: the UK's biggest issue [editorial]. *Lancet*, **349**, 1185.

Bartley M (2004). *Health inequality: an introduction to theories, concepts and methods*. Polity Press, Cambridge.

Benzeval M, Judge K and Whitehead M (1995). *Tackling inequalities in health; an agenda for action*. King's Fund, London.

Bond FW and Bunce D (2001). Job control mediates change in a work reorganization intervention for stress reduction. *Journal of Occupational Health Psychology*, **6**, 290–302.

Burström B, Whitehead M, Lindholm C and Diderichsen F (2000). Inequality in the social consequences of illness: how well do people with long-term illness fare in the British and Swedish labor markets? *International Journal of Health Services*, **30**, 435–51.

Cavelaars AEJM, Kunst AE, Geurts JJM *et al.* (1998a). Morbidity differences by occupational class among men in seven European countries: an application of the Erikson Goldthorpe social class scheme. *International Journal of Epidemiology*, **27**, 222–30.

Cavelaars AEJM, Kunst AE, Geurts JJM *et al.* (1998b). Differences in self-reported morbidity by educational level: a comparison of 11 Western European countries. *Journal of Epidemiology and Community Health*, **52**, 219–27.

Cavelaars AEJM, Kunst AE, Geurts JJM *et al.* (2000). Educational differences in smoking: international comparison. *British Medical Journal*, **320**, 1102–7.

Cavelaars AEJM, Kunst AE and Mackenbach JP (1997). Socio-economic differences in risk-factors for morbidity and mortality in the European Community. An international comparison. *Journal of Health Psychology*, **2**, 353–72.

Chauvin P and Lebas J (eds.) (1998). *Précarité et Santé*. Flammarion, Paris.

Costa G and Faggiano F (eds.) (1994). *L'equità nella salute in Italia*. Fondazione Smith Kline, Franco Angeli, Milan.

Costa G, Spadea T and Dirindin N (2002). Italy. In: J Mackenbach and M Bakker (eds) *Reducing inequalities in health: a European perspective*. Routledge, London.

Dahlgren G and Whitehead M (1992). *Policies and strategies to promote equity in health*. World Health Organization, Copenhagen.

Dalstra JAA, Kunst AE, Borrell C *et al.* (2005). Socio-economic differences in the prevalence of common chronic diseases: an overview of eight European countries. *International Journal of Epidemiology* **34**, 316–26.

Davey Smith G, Blane D and Bartley M (1994). Explanations for socio-economic differentials in mortality. Evidence from Britain and elsewhere. *European Journal of Public Health*, **4**, 131–44.

Davey Smith G, Ebrahim S and Frankel S (2001). How policy informs the evidence. *British Medical Journal*, **322**, 184–5.

Davey Smith G, Morris JN and Shaw M (1998). The Independent Inquiry into Inequalities in Health [editorial]. *British Medical Journal*, **317**, 1465–6.

Department of Health (1995). *Variations in health: what can the Department of Health and the NHS do? Variations Sub-Group of the Chief Medical Officers Health of the Nation Working Group*. The Stationery Office, London.

Department of Health (1999a). *Saving lives: our healthier nation*. Stationery Office, London.

Department of Health (1999b). *Reducing health inequalities: an action report*. Stationery Office, London.

Department of Health (2001). *From vision to reality*. Stationery Office, London.

Department of Health (2004). *Choosing health: making healthy choices easier*. Stationery Office, London.

Doorslaer E van, Wagstaff A, van der Burg H *et al.* (2000). Equity in the delivery of health care in Europe and the US. *J Health Econ*, **19**, 553–83.

Droomers M, Schrijvers CTM and Mackenbach JP (2002). Why do lower educated people continue smoking? Explanations from the longitudinal GLOBE study. *Health Psychology*, **21**, 263–72.

Eccles M, Grimshaw J, Campbell M and Ramsay C (2003). Research designs for studies evaluating the effectiveness of change and improvement strategies. *Quality and Safety in Health Care*, **3**, 47–52.

Elm E von and Egger M (2004). The scandal of poor epidemiological research. *British Medical Journal*, **329**, 868–9.

Ford G, Ecob R, Hunt K, MacIntyre S and West P (1994). Patterns of class inequality in health through the lifespan – class gradients at 15, 35 and 55 years in the West of Scotland. *Social Science and Medicine*, **39**, 1037–50.

Gaunt-Richardson P, Amos A, Howie G, McKie L and Moore M (1999). *Women, low income and smoking – breaking down the barriers*. ASH Scotland/Health Education Board for Scotland, Edinburgh.

Grabauskas V and Padaiga Z (2002). Lithuania. In J: Mackenbach and M Bakker (eds) *Reducing inequalities in health: a European perspective*. Routledge, London.

GRADE Working Group (2004). Grading quality of evidence and strength of recommendations. *British Medical Journal*, **328**, 1490–7.

HM Treasury (1998). *Comprehensive spending review: cross-departmental review of provision for young children*. Supporting papers, vol. 1 and 2. Stationery Office, London.

Huisman M, Kunst AE, Andersen O *et al.* (2004). Socioeconomic inequalities in mortality among elderly people in 11 European populations. *Journal of Epidemiology and Community Health*, **58**, 468–75.

Huisman M, Kunst AE, Bopp M *et al.* (2005). Educational inequalities in cause-specific mortality in middle-aged and older men and women in eight western European populations. *Lancet*, **365**, 493–500.

Huisman M, Kunst AE and Mackenbach JP (2003). Socioeconomic inequalities in morbidity among the elderly; a European overview. *Social Science and Medicine*, **57**, 861–73.

Huisman M, Kunst AE and Mackenbach JP (2005). Educational inequalities in smoking among men and women aged 16 years and older in eleven European countries. *Tobacco Control*, **14**, 106–13.

Kuijer PP, Visser B and Kemper HC (1999). Job rotation as a factor in reducing physical workload at a refuse collecting department. *Ergonomics*, **42**, 1167–78.

Kunst AE, Groenhof F, Mackenbach JP and the EU Working Group on Socioeconomic Inequalities in Health (1998a). Mortality by occupational class among men 30–64 years in 11 European countries. *Social Science and Medicine*, **46**, 1459–76.

Kunst AE, Groenhof F, Mackenbach JP and the EU Working Group on Socioeconomic Inequalities in Health (1998b). Occupational class and cause-specific mortality in middle-aged men in 11 European countries: a comparison of population-based studies. *British Medical Journal*, **316**, 1636–41.

Kunst AE (1997). *Cross-national comparisons of socio-economic differences in mortality*. PhD-thesis. Erasmus University Rotterdam.

Lang T, Nicaud V, Darne B and Rueff B (1995). Improving hypertension control among excessive alcohol drinkers: a randomised controlled trial in France. The WALPA Group. *Journal of Epidemiology and Community Health*, **49**, 610–16.

Lang T, Nicaud V, Slama K, *et al.* (2000). Smoking cessation at the workplace. Results of a randomised controlled intervention study. Worksite physicians from the AIREL group. *Journal of Epidemiology and Community Health*, **54**, 349–54.

Leclerc A, Fassin D, Grandjean H, Kaminski M and Lang T (eds.) (2000). *Les inégalités sociales de santé*. La Découverte, Paris.

Lynch JW, Davey Smith G, Kaplan GA and House JS (2000). Income inequality and mortality: importance to health of individual income, psychosocial environment, or material conditions. *British Medical Journal*, **320**, 1200–4.

Lynch JW, Kaplan GA and Salonen JT (1997). Why do poor people behave poorly? Variation in adult health behaviours and psychosocial characteristics by stages of the socio-economic life course. *Social Science and Medicine*, **44**, 809–19.

Macintyre S (1997). The Black Report and beyond: what are the issues? *Social Science and Medicine*, **44**, 723–45.

Macintyre S (2003). Evidence-based policy making. *British Medical Journal*, **326**, 5–6.

Macintyre S, Chalmers I, Horton R and Smith R (2001). Using evidence to inform health policy: case study. *British Medical Journal*, **322**, 222–5.

Mackenbach J and Bakker M (eds) (2002). *Reducing inequalities in health: a European perspective*. Routledge, London.

Mackenbach JP, Bakker MJ and the European Network on Interventions and Policies to Reduce Inequalities in Health (2003a). Tackling socio-economic inequalities in health: an analysis of recent European experiences. *Lancet*, **362**, 1409–14.

Mackenbach JP, Bos V, Andersen O *et al.* (2003b). Widening socio-economic inequalities in mortality in six western European countries. *International Journal of Epidemiology*, **32**, 830–7.

Mackenbach JP, Cavelaars AEJM, Kunst AE, Groenhof F and the EU Working Group on Socioeconomic Inequalities in Health (2000). Socioeconomic inequalities in cardiovascular disease mortality: an international study. *European Heart Journal*, **21**, 1141–51.

Mackenbach JP and Gunning-Schepers LJ (1997). How should interventions to reduce inequalities in health be evaluated? *Journal of Epidemiology and Community Health*, **51**, 359–64.

Mackenbach JP, Huisman M, Andersen O *et al.* (2004). Inequalities in lung cancer mortality by the educational level in 10 European populations. *European Journal of Cancer*, **40**, 126–35.

Mackenbach JP, Kunst AE, Cavelaars AEJM, Groenhof F, Geurts JJM and the EU Working Group on Socioeconomic Inequalities in Health (1997). Socioeconomic inequalities in morbidity and mortality in Western Europe. *Lancet*, **349**, 1655–9.

Mackenbach JP, Kunst AE, Groenhof F *et al.* (1999). Socioeconomic inequalities in mortality among women and among men: an international study. *American Journal of Public Health*, **89**, 1800–6.

Mackenbach JP and Stronks K (2002). A strategy for tackling health inequalities in the Netherlands. *British Medical Journal*, **325**, 1029–32.

Mackenbach JP and Stronks K (2004). The development of a strategy for tackling health inequalities in the Netherlands. *International Journal for Equity in Health*, **3**, 11–17.

Mackenbach JP, van de Mheen H and Stronks K (1994). A prospective cohort study investigating the explanation of socio-economic inequalities in health in The Netherlands. *Social Science and Medicine*, **38**, 299–308.

Marmot MG, Davey Smith G, Stansfeld S *et al.* (1991) Health inequalities among British civil servants: The Whitehall II study. *Lancet*, **337**, 1387–93.

Marmot MG and Wilkinson RG (eds.) (1999). *Social determinants of health*. Oxford University Press, Oxford.

Mielck A, Graham H and Bremberg S (2002). Children, an important target group for the reduction of socio-economic inequalities in health. In: J Mackenbach J and M Bakker (eds) *Reducing inequalities in health: a European perspective*. Routledge, London.

Ministry of Health and Social Affairs (1991). *Concerning public health issues* (Government Bill 1990/91:175). Norstedts Förlag, Stockholm.

Ministry of Health and Social Affairs, Stockholm (2000) Hälsa på lika villkor – nationella mål för folkhälsan. Slutbetänkande av nationella folkhälsokommittén (*Health on equal terms – final proposal on national targets for public health*). Ministry of Health and Social Affairs, Stockholm. (SOU 2000:91).

Ministry of Social Affairs and Health Helsinki (1986). *Health for All by the year 2000*. Helsinki.

Navarro V, Benach J and the Scientific Commission for the study of health inequalities in Spain (1996). *Social inequalities in health in Spain*. Ministerio de Sanidad y Consumo, Madrid.

Oliver MA (2001). Health inequalities policy: do we need evidence on effectiveness? [letter to the editor]. BMJ.com (rapid responses to: Davey Smith G, Ebrahim S, Frankel S). How policy informs the evidence. *British Medical Journal*, **322**, 1849–1850.

Petticrew M, Whitehead M, Macintyre SJ, Graham H and Egan M (2004). Evidence for public health policy on inequalities I: The reality according to policy-makers. *Journal of Epidemiology and Community Health*, **58**, 811–16.

Prättälä R, Berg MA, Puska P (1992). Diminishing or increasing contrasts? Social class variation in Finnish food consumption patterns 1979–1990. *European Journal of Clinical Nutritition*, **42** (Suppl.), 16–20.

Programmacommissie Sociaal-economische gezondheidsverschillen (1994) *Onderzoeksprogramma sociaal-economische gezondheidsverschillen; eindverslag en aanbevelingen*. Ministerie van WVC, Rijswijk.

Programmacommissie Sociaal-Economische GezondheidsVerschillen-tweede fase. (2001) Sociaal-economische gezondheidsverschillen verkleinen. Eindrapportage en beleidsaanbevelingen van de Programmacommissie SEGV-II. (*Reducing socio-economic inequalities in health. Final report and policy recommendations of the Programme Committee SEIH-II*). ZorgOnderzoek Nederland, Den Haag.

Roberts H (2000). What is Sure Start? *Archive of Disease in Childhood*, **82**, 435–7.

Schrijvers CTM, Stronks K, Mheen H, van de and Mackenbach JP (1999). Explaining educational differences in mortality: the role of behavioral and material factors. *American Journal of Public Health*, **89**, 535–40.

Sorgdrager J, Matthesius DM, Groothoff JW, de Haan J and Post D (2001). Een dokteres in de praktijk; effecten van een praktijkverpleegkundige op de zorg voor patiënten met astma/COPD. In: K Stronks (ed) *Sociaal-economische gezondheidsverschillen: van verklaren naar verkleinen, deel 4*. Zorgonderzoek Nederland, The Hague.

Stronks K and Hulshof J (eds) (2001). *De kloof verkleinen*. Van Gorcum, Assen.

Syme SL (1989). Control and health: a personal perspective. In: A Steptoe and A Appels (eds) *Stress, personal control, and health*. Wiley, London.

Thomson H, Hoskins R, Petticrew M *et al*. (2004). Evaluating the health effects of social interventions. *British Medical Journal*, **328**, 282–5.

Tountas Y, Karnaki P and Triantafyllou D (2002). Greece. In: J Mackenbach and M Bakker (eds) *Reducing inequalities in health: a European perspective*. Routledge, London.

Townsend P and Davidson N (1992). The Black Report 1982. In: P Townsend, M Whitehead M and N Davidson (eds) *Inequalities in health: The Black Report and the health divide*, pp. 209–213. Penguin Books, London.

Vågerö D and Illsley R (1995). Explaining health inequalities: beyond Black and Barker. *European Sociological Review*, **3**, 1–23.

van Doorslaer E, Wagstaff A, Bleichrodt H *et al*. (1997). Income-related inequalities in health: some international comparisons. *Health Economy*, **16**, 93–112.

Wallerstein N (2002). Empowerment to reduce health disparities. *Scandinavian Journal of Public Health*, (Suppl.) **59**, 72–77.

Website: http://www.kttl.helsinki.fi/projektit/Helsinki/helsinkistudy.htm

Whitehead M and Dahlgren G (1991). What can be done about inequalities in health? *Lancet*, **338**, 1059–63.

Whitehead M, Petticrew M, Graham H, Macintyre SJ, Bambra C, Egan M (2004). Evidence for public health policy on inequalities II: Assembling the evidence jigsaw. *Journal Epidemiology and Community Health*, **58**, 817–21.

Whitehead M (1998). Diffusion of ideas on social inequalities in health: a European perspective. *Millbank Quarterly*, **76**, 469–92.

Whitehead M (1992). The health divide. In: P Townsend , M Whitehead, N Davidson, (eds) *Inequalities in health: The Black Report and the health divide*, pp. 215–450. Penguin Books, London.

World Health Organization (1985). *Targets for health for all*. WHO, Copenhagen.

Index